RY
ON E1 2AD

A guide for doctors

**Ruth Chambers
Gill Wakley
Steve Field
and
Simon Ellis**

**Foreword by
David Graham**

RADCLIFFE MEDICAL PRESS

Radcliffe Medical Press Ltd
18 Marcham Road
Abingdon
Oxon OX14 1AA
United Kingdom

www.radcliffe-oxford.com
The Radcliffe Medical Press electronic catalogue and online ordering facility.
Direct sales to anywhere in the world.

British Library Cataloguing in Publication Data

A catalogue record for this book is available from the British Library.

ISBN 1 85775 982 6

Typeset by Advance Typesetting Ltd, Oxfordshire
Printed and bound by TJ International Ltd, Padstow, Cornwall

Contents

Foreword

I am delighted to be asked to provide the foreword for this excellent book. The timing of its publication could not be better. This practical and informative guide will be of value to doctors working in both primary and secondary care.

Doctors should not be apprehensive about appraisal, but should see the benefits and welcome its introduction. Appraisal is a positive process, which is of value to the doctor, the organisation and, ultimately, the patient. We should embrace appraisal and use it to develop and drive good practice. As Ruth, Gill, Steve and Simon point out, appraisal should be used to plan and formulate its important output – the personal development plan (PDP). The plan should be agreed and achievable and will assist the doctor and the organisation. The PDP will then form the basis of the next appraisal. Appraisal should not be viewed as being regulatory, but should be seen as being developmental.

Appraisal is separate, but closely linked, to revalidation and it is anticipated that revalidation will be formally introduced in the near future. A robust appraisal process pulling together the required information will provide the evidence for revalidation.

In this book the authors have put together a practical guide to assist doctors with appraisal that, hopefully, will remove some of the anxieties and allay fears. The book covers appraisal for all doctors and uses appropriate examples which show how appraisal can be implemented and used in the 'real' world. Examples of good practice will help to develop the process, and the book covers the whole of the appraisal process, including the difficult areas and specific situations, for example appraisal for doctors in academic medicine and the introduction of the Follett reforms.

The book displays a good balance between appropriate educational theory and, most importantly, the practicalities of carrying out and implementing appraisal.

I, like the authors, remain convinced that appraisal should be viewed in a positive light and *Appraisal for the Apprehensive* makes a valuable contribution detailing the background and framework for evaluation, successfully combining some educational theory with practical advice which should allay any misplaced concerns. Appraisal is here to help the profession and the patient.

Good luck.

David Graham
Postgraduate Dean, Mersey Deanery
Chair, Appraisal Implementation Group
October 2002

About the authors

Ruth Chambers BM BS, BMed Sci, DRCOG, Cert Med Ed, FRCGP, DM has been a GP for 20 years. Her previous experience has encompassed a wide range of research and educational activities, including stress and the health of doctors, the quality of healthcare, healthy working, teenagers' sexual health and many other topics. She is currently a part-time GP and the Professor of Primary Care Development at the School of Health, Staffordshire University. She was the Chairman of Staffordshire Medical Audit Advisory Group for three years until 1996. She was a GP trainer for four years. Ruth has initiated and run all types of educational initiatives and activities for health professionals and managers. Ruth runs appraiser training courses for doctors and other health professionals.

Gill Wakley MB ChB, MFFP, MIPM, MD started in general practice in 1966, but transferred to community medicine shortly afterwards and then into public health. A desire for increased contact with patients caused a move back into general practice, together with community gynaecology. She has been combining the two, in varying amounts, ever since. Gill has been heavily involved in learning and teaching throughout. She worked in a training general practice, became an instructing doctor and a regional assessor in family planning, and was until recently a Senior Clinical Lecturer with the Primary Care Department at Keele University. Like Ruth, she has run all types of educational initiatives and activities, from individual mentoring and instruction to small-group work, plenary lectures, workshops and courses for a wide range of health professionals and lay people.

Steve Field MB ChB, DRCOG, MMEd, ILTM, FRCGP is Regional Postgraduate Medical Dean, West Midlands Deanery, Honorary Professor of Medical Education at the University of Warwick and Chairman of the Education Network, Royal College of General Practitioners. He has been a GP since 1986 and continues to work part-time at Bellevue Medical Centre in inner-city Birmingham. For many years he was an examiner and member of the Royal College of General Practitioners' examination board. He has also been vice-chair of the Committee of GP Education Directors (COGPED), chair of the Implementation Committee for the UK GP Registrar Scheme and chair of the National Summative Assessment Board for General Practice. Steve continues to be actively involved in teaching and learning with particular interest in communication skills and assessment methodologies.

Simon Ellis MA, MB, BChir, FRCP, MD is a Consultant Neurologist at North Stafford-shire Hospital and was formally a lecturer in Neurology at Oxford University. He is the Visiting Professor in Neurosciences at Staffordshire University and has several years of experience of running teaching sessions on appraisal as part of 'Teaching the Teachers' courses. Simon is Clinical Director of the Directorate of Neurosciences at the North Staffordshire Hospital.

PART 1

All about appraisal

1

Appraisal: an introduction

'**Appraisal** is an official or formal evaluation of the strengths and weaknesses of someone or something.'

(*Collins COBUILD English Dictionary*, 1999)

Appraisal is a formative and developmental process which is being introduced by the Department of Health for all general practitioner principals and hospital consultants working in the NHS across the UK. While the details of the appraisal system will vary for consultants and GPs and for each of the home countries, the educational principles remain the same. The aims of the appraisal system are to give doctors regular feedback on their previous and continuing performance and identify educational and developmental needs.

The aim of this book is to help you to gain a better understanding of appraisal so that you can get the most out of the process.

The drive to introduce formal appraisals came initially as part of the programme to introduce clinical governance across the NHS as laid out in the 1998 consultation document *A First Class Service*.[1] Momentum was gained with the publication of *Supporting Doctors, Protecting Patients* (1999) which outlined a set of proposals to help prevent doctors in England developing problems.[2] Appraisal was at the heart of the proposals. This consultation document advocated the introduction of appraisal as 'a positive process to give someone feedback on their performance, to chart their continuing progress and to identify development needs. It is a forward looking process essential for the developmental and educational planning needs of an individual. Assessment is the process of measuring progress against agreed criteria ... It is not the primary aim of appraisal to scrutinise doctors to see if they are performing poorly but rather to help them consolidate and improve on good performance aiming towards excellence.' The document went on to suggest that appraisal should be made comprehensive and compulsory for doctors working in the NHS and form part of a future revalidation system.

The Department of Health in England expects that important areas to cover in appraisal include actions to:

- maintain skills and level of service to patients
- develop or acquire new skills
- change or improve existing practice.

In addition, the appraisal should also address other areas of particular importance to the individual doctor. A standardised approach has been developed which utilises approved documentation. This should ensure that information from a variety of NHS employers is recorded consistently. The format of the paperwork is slightly different for consultants and GPs.

Consultant appraisal was formally introduced in April 2001, while appraisal for GPs became a contractual requirement in April 2002. It is hoped that appraisal will be extended quickly to involve doctors from non-consultant career grades, GP non-principals and locums. Appraisal systems for junior doctors, which include GP registrars, are being developed to complement existing formative assessment and record of in-training assessment (RITA) systems.

Appraisal must be a positive, formative and developmental process to support high-quality patient care and improve clinical standards. Appraisal is different from but linked to revalidation.[3] Revalidation is the process whereby doctors will be regularly required to demonstrate that they are fit to practise. Appraisal feeds into this by contributing to the evidence that a doctor submits into the revalidation process. Appraisal will provide the regular structured recording system for documenting progress towards revalidation and identifying needs as part of the doctor's personal development plan. Both the NHS appraisal and the revalidation structures are based on the same seven headings set out in the General Medical Council's (GMC's) guidance *Good Medical Practice*.[4] The GMC claims, therefore, that most of the evidence for revalidation requirements should be available from the material produced for appraisal. In this way they can be seen as complementary procedures, as illustrated in Figure 1.1.

The introduction of appraisal to a hospital department, health centre or GP practice could be perceived as a threat but, done well, appraisal is empowering and yields many benefits to the doctor, to the health service and ultimately to the care of our patients.

Appraisal is a real opportunity to motivate doctors – and judging by what you read about the morale of doctors in the medical press, motivation and positive vibes are just what is needed! Appraisal is not an adversarial system; it is an opportunity to support and praise the appraisee. A well-conducted appraisal will help doctors form an objective view of their past performance and help them to improve and take on greater responsibility in the future.

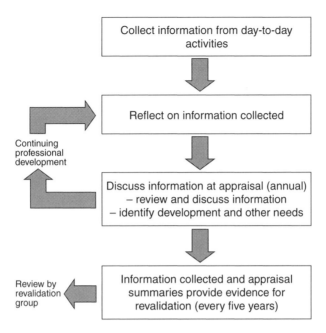

Figure 1.1: The appraisal and revalidation process.[3]

The success of any clinical service is determined to a great extent by the performance of its human resource – the people working in the department or practice or elsewhere in the NHS. The same can be said of successful businesses which have been involved in appraisal systems for many years. The business needs information about its staff concerning their performance in the job, their future potential, and their education, training and development needs. The individuals need to know what is expected of them, how they are perceived to have performed, how they are valued as members of the team and whether there is anything they could do to improve their performance or to develop their careers. Senior managers, including chief executives, are appraised in successful businesses – so an empowering appraisal in the clinical setting should also reap benefits for the individual and the health service as a whole.

Our business is the National Health Service. The introduction of appraisal should help the business become even more successful by helping doctors to consolidate and improve on their good performance while identifying areas where further development may be necessary. Appraisal is, however, a two-way process: not only will time and resources be needed to make the appraisal systems a success, but appraisal will also identify issues that will require additional investment by the NHS in the educational and organisational infrastructure.

> **Box 1.1:**
>
> The chief executive of the British Association of Medical Managers (BAMM),
> Dr Jenny Simpson, believes that appraisal will come to have a central place
> in improving quality. 'We are talking about a process that will be at the core of
> clinical governance and revalidation. It has to be more than a snapshot of how
> people are performing on a particular day – it has to be robust and look at the
> effectiveness of an individual's clinical practice.'[5,6]

The successful appraisal process should be empowering; it should motivate
and guide the individual. It should result in the production of a personal development plan (PDP) because appraisal is concerned with setting personal
learning goals.[7,8] It should also contribute to the wider practice or hospital
department professional development plans, to the broader development
plans for the hospital or primary care organisation and ultimately to the
national agenda via health improvement and modernisation plans (HIMPs).

Appraisal and revalidation are here to stay. Choice is not an option. Reading this book should help you to gain a greater understanding of the processes
involved to be able to approach appraisal in a positive and constructive way.
Then you should be able to take advantage of what you will begin to recognise
is a system designed to help you and your patients.

References

1   Department of Health (1998) *A First Class Service*. Department of Health, London.

2   Department of Health (1999) *Supporting Doctors, Protecting Patients*. Department
of Health, London.

3   General Medical Council (2002) *The Guide to Appraisal and Revalidation*.
www.revalidationuk.info (accessed June 2002).

4   General Medical Council (2001) *Good Medical Practice*. General Medical Council,
London.

5   Moore A (2001) Turned to good account. In: M Crail (ed.) *Leadership in the NHS*.
Health Service Journal, London.

6   British Association of Medical Managers (1999) *Appraisal in Action*. British
Association of Medical Managers, Stockport.

7   Wakley G, Chambers R and Field S (2000) *Continuing Professional Development in
Primary Care: making it happen*. Radcliffe Medical Press, Oxford.

8   Rughani A (2000) *The GP's Guide to Personal Development Plans*. Radcliffe Medical
Press, Oxford.

2

Preparing for an appraisal

Effective appraisal is a positive, formative and developmental process designed to support high-quality patient care and improve clinical standards. While the structured format is slightly different for hospital consultants and GPs, the educational principles and the preparation needed are the same.

The secret to preparing for an appraisal is to collect evidence about the standards of your practice throughout the year, so that you do yourself justice and are not forced to throw information together about various aspects of your work in a last-minute rush.

Effective appraisal depends on both the appraiser and you, as the appraisee, preparing for the appraisal interview in advance. There should be an opportunity for you to exchange information and documents before the interview. The appraiser should understand the pressures that the demands of patient care and limited resources create. He or she should be able to make allowances for any issues or problems that you have had in your everyday work that are beyond your control. You need to collect facts about any such pressures or resource problems, rather than impressions. Be specific rather than whinge. Then your evidence regarding the barriers to you and other colleagues achieving best practice can be collated to inform business planning, the workforce and the educational strategies of your primary care organisation or hospital trust.

Box 2.1: Consultants and GPs are being appraised using very similar structures

1 Personal details.
2 Details of current medical activities.
3 Good medical practice.
    3.1 Good medical care.
    3.2 Maintaining good medical practice.
    3.3 Working relationships with colleagues.
    3.4 Relations with patients.
    3.5 Teaching and training.
    3.6 Probity.

continued overleaf

> 3.7   Health.
> 3.8   Any other points.
> 4   Management activity.
> 5   Research.
> 6   Report on development action in the last year.
> 7   Summary of appraisal discussion with agreed action and personal develop-
>   ment plan.

Become an appraiser yourself?

A really good way to prepare is to be trained as an appraiser yourself and
undertake appraisals with other doctors. Then you will know what sort of
level and range of performance you are expected to cover within the scope of
an appraisal, and you will learn a lot from the way others approach appraisal
and undertake their subsequent action plans.

Alternatively, or additionally, you could contribute to other people's
appraisals, such as those of nursing or manager colleagues, and learn from
your close contact with their 'official' appraisers.

Anticipate the appraisal forms that you will be required to complete

It is important to ensure that you understand the appraisal paperwork requirements because the formats for GPs and consultants are slightly different.
Box 2.1 summarises the section headings. It is worth logging on to the website
www.revalidationuk.info because it contains all of the up-to-date information
available for both groups. You might want to use an electronic version once it
is available (www.appraisals.nhs.uk). Use the standardised paperwork rather
than invent your own version, as the Department of Health wants information to be recorded and expressed in a consistent manner, year on year, and
between individual doctors.

See Appendix 2 for examples of the documentation for general practitioners
and hospital consultants in England.

If you record your personal and professional development throughout the
year under the same headings required for the appraisal, you should avoid
unnecessary work in preparing your appraisal folder and rearranging the
information and evidence that you have gathered for other purposes.

Box 2.2:

'One thing we have learnt is that it is far better to collect your evidence for the appraisal process over the course of the year than to try to find it just before a session is booked ... Certainly where this has been done rigorously, it makes the appraisal process very efficient and straightforward' (hospital consultant).[1]

It will take considerable time to complete the required appraisal forms. Allow at least four hours, and even more time than this if you know that you are not good at completing forms, or if you have had little previous experience of preparing for such a review and assessment of your work.

Completing the appraisal paperwork

Some sections of the forms may seem irrelevant to your individual circumstances – as, for instance, you may not be involved with research, or have little interest in, or responsibility for, management. You should just comment in these sorts of sections in a few words. However, you may realise, from looking through the later chapters in Part 2 of this book, that you do more of these activities and are able to write more about your work in these areas than you had thought at first.

Box 2.3:

Dr Rural thought she would have to leave blank the section on teaching and training. She could never get a locum in her isolated area, so she rarely attended any outside activities and thought that her general practice was unsuitable for training. Then she realised that the nurses frequently turned to her for information on medical conditions, and that she went into the local school and to youth groups to talk about health matters. So she could ask the nurses, youth workers and school teachers for their feedback and evaluation of those teaching activities and fill in that section of the paperwork after all.

The material you include in your appraisal paperwork should describe the important facts, features, themes and issues of your work. You should reflect upon the entire span of your work as a doctor within and outside the NHS. The factual basis of the information you collect as you progress through the year should help your reflections to be accurate, rather than present the rosy picture that you recall when looking back over time.

Do not repeat the same information unnecessarily in different sections of the forms. Be as brief or as lengthy in your responses as is appropriate to the information that you have to convey – but try to keep to the point. Your appraiser will be looking for evidence of your assertions in the supporting documentation and through discussion with you.

The papers you assemble in support of a completed form should be listed in the relevant spaces on the particular pages. Compile the documents as a folder, organised in the same order as the section headings appear in the official appraisal paperwork. If the same material is listed in the form more than once to illustrate or justify different information, do not duplicate it within your appraisal folder but describe or cross-reference where it can be found in the previous or subsequent sections of the appraisal form.

Triangulation

One methodology frequently used in the social sciences (and by the Commission of Health Improvement [CHI] visiting inspection teams) is triangulation. If you have three pieces of evidence pointing in a particular direction then it is probably true. One of the ways of helping you to organise your own thoughts and direct the appraiser in the direction you want him or her to go is to use an evidence table. Table 2.1 gives an example of an evidence table from a consultant's portfolio structuring the evidence about his research activity.

Table 2.1:

Area	Evidence	Linkage
1 Research	Honorary Senior Clinical Lecturer in School of Postgraduate Medicine	Demonstrates academic affiliation
	List of publications	Demonstrates research active
	Selected publications	Demonstrates some publications of quality

Lead the appraisal in the direction you want it to go. If you arrive at the appraisal with two box files and a carrier bag of papers and expect the appraiser to sort through it for evidence of your good practice – think again. You have just demonstrated your contempt for the appraisal process and that you are lacking in organisational skills.

Subverting the process

Appraisal, as originally conceived, is not a performance management tool. It is a developmental tool, to help the individual to develop, professionally and educationally. The government has confused appraisal with performance management and has linked it to revalidation. The medical profession in the UK is going to have to spend time and energy on the appraisal process, so it is in our interest to make it work to our best advantage. Doctors are intelligent, shrewd creatures and it is not beyond the wit of most of us to subvert the process of appraisal back to its original intent to that of a developmental tool. Using appraisal to help individuals rather than to chastise them will bring out the best in them and, perversely, be more likely to achieve the government's aim of improving the quality of medical care in the UK.

Moving from appraisals to revalidation

Appraisal and revalidation will be based largely on the same sources of information – presented in the same structure as the headings set out in the GMC guidance in *Good Medical Practice*. The two processes perform different functions. Whereas revalidation involves an assessment against a standard of fitness to practise medicine, appraisal is concerned with the doctor's professional development within his or her working environment and the needs of the organisation for which the doctor works. We cannot be sure exactly what information the GMC will require you to submit for revalidation until the pilots have been completed and the final regulations are published. We expect that revalidation of doctors' professional qualifications will start in 2004–05 and that those being revalidated will be asked to include copies of their folders and appraisers' reports from their annual appraisals from 2001–02 or, as years go by, from the previous five years.

Box 2.4: Extent of evidence for revalidation

The uncertainty about the extent of evidence that will be required for revalidation is reflected in the following quote from a member of the General Practitioners Committee (GPC). 'Appraisal as it has been agreed by the GPC is about the sincere engagement of GPs in a formative process. Relying on five formative appraisals by themselves may not be enough and the external quality assurance of revalidation might involve inspection of the evidence of the quality of practice e.g. audits.'

On the other hand, some are reassured. 'Now that it has become clear that revalidation by the GMC will be based on a series of completed appraisals, this should also be a very straightforward and painless process' (hospital consultant).[1]

Making the most of the appraisal process

You could approach your appraisal with fear and trepidation, or you could resolve to be positive and put your trust into the process and the appraiser, and make the system work for you. You should expect a fair hearing from another doctor who is familiar with your medical specialty and who has been trained to carry out appraisal. In general practice, being 'credible with peers' is an essential feature of the person specification that primary care organisations are directed to use when selecting appraisers.

If you do not believe that appraisal will be a meaningful process in which you can trust the medical colleague who will be appraising your work, you may be driven to conceal particular areas where your work or performance is imperfect. If this happens, your personal development plan (PDP) would be meaningless as you may prioritise areas to learn more about that build entirely on your strengths rather than addressing your weaknesses.

Box 2.5:

'I am looking forward to my appraisal to have the opportunity to reflect in a constructive way about what I do with a colleague I trust' (hospital consultant).

Hospital trusts and primary care organisations are expected to take action as far as possible to address the educational and developmental needs of consultants, GPs and other doctors, as well as the service development requirements identified and agreed in the course of appraisal. Therefore appraisal should provide an opportunity to harness your organisation's support for your development needs.

As long as you, and the appraiser backed by the trust or primary care organisation, collect *facts* rather than unsubstantiated opinions, the appraisal exercise should be fair. One way to be sure that the information is fair is to collect it from a broad base of sources or informants – so consider adopting 360° feedback from junior and senior colleagues about your performance, and doing the same for them (*see* page 109 for more information about 360° feedback).[2,3]

Some of the consultants working at Glenfield Hospital Trust (*see* Box 2.6) are keen on 360° assessment with views being sought from peers, line managers and juniors. Consultants are encouraged to collect the information themselves and then discuss it with their appraisers. Evidence about their clinical work can come from a variety of sources – audit, information about volume of work done, outcomes etc. – and the appraisal can also cover subjects such as how medical students view their teaching or communication with patients.[4]

Box 2.6:   Upping the ante: Glenfield Hospital Trust[4]

The Glenfield scheme was introduced gradually over three years, beginning with simply reviewing consultants' job plans and then developing that process into a relatively informal appraisal system. Consultants are appraised annually by their clinical director. The appraisal interview usually takes between an hour and an hour-and-a-half and covers a review of the components of the job: personal 'needs' required to do the job such as additional equipment or staff; personal and professional training plans; individual performance assessment; and objective setting, which can be in any field but has to be capable of producing measurable achievements. It covers all aspects of a consultant's work. Any major problems with consultants' work should be picked up and tackled as they arise rather than waiting for an annual appraisal. The system is not linked to disciplinary action, but some minor problems with consultants' work have been picked up and addressed as a result of the appraisal system.

Doctors' fears about the appraisal process

Common fears that doctors have about appraisal seem to centre around:

- uncertainty about what the process will involve
- a lack of confidence in the skills of the appraiser
- reluctance to reveal weaknesses about their practice or performance in case they are penalised in some way
- the time taken in preparing for and undertaking the appraisal
- the lack of resources for professional development
- the lack of resources to remedy deficits in service delivery.

The effects of a personality clash between the appraiser and the doctor being appraised may well affect the conduct of the appraisal discussion and the appraiser's subsequent report. If the appraiser lacks interpersonal and facilitation skills, this may lead to the appraiser dominating the discussion, so that the appraisee does not make a meaningful contribution and lacks ownership of the objectives in his or her personal development plan.

An appraiser's lack of expertise or experience in education may lead to the appraiser giving feedback that is too vague to be useful to the person being appraised, or even worse, may demotivate or humiliate that person. An appraiser may irritate the person being appraised by ignoring that person's preferred style of learning, indicating a lack of rapport between them. An overbearing appraiser may urge the appraisee to 'be like me' rather than enable the appraisee to follow his or her own chosen path of professional development. Alternatively, an appraiser might adopt an overly reflective manner that may annoy appraisees who observe this 'textbook' behaviour. It is fruitless to use techniques such as mirroring or echoing what the appraisee has just said as a way of encouragement, or to use silence to try to force an appraisee to speak, if the doctor being appraised prefers direct interchange of factual information. Adopting a tried and tested technique from management training in an uncritical manner may also be counterproductive if the person being appraised dislikes such an approach.

Box 2.7:   Example of an appraisal where the appraiser tries to humiliate the appraisee

Anonymised extracts from recent appraisal of Drew who works for Social Services

Achievement of objectives

Drew produces thorough, detailed and readable reports, but Drew's report turnaround time continues to be too long. He recognises this is a problem and he will need to make further efforts to work on this in the current year.

   Drew has made some progress on the use of IT and now manages some of his emails when he is in the office. As methodologies increasingly rely on electronic transfer of information and office systems require computer literacy, Drew recognises that this is an area he will need to continue to work on.

Working with others

Drew recognises that he needs to be constantly aware of the effect that his irrepressible humour has on others, so that he remains sensitive to their feelings and their ability to contribute to group business.

Personal effectiveness

Drew is a good communicator, particularly verbally, and prefers to rely on those skills rather than the use of visual aids such as PowerPoint.

Doctors' reluctance to reveal any areas of underperformance in their practice is partly because they mistrust how others working outside the situation under discussion may interpret the information. They fear the unfair apportioning of blame for underperformance to individuals rather than the organisation, when patient load and associated limitations on resources affect the standards of care. The quotes from consultants in Box 2.8 illustrate their hostility to appraisal.

Box 2.8:

'If someone does their job you don't need appraisal' (psychiatrist).

'Appraisal is an opportunity for someone to criticise your work if you are not doing your job' (general surgeon).

Information that is used by the hospital trust or primary care organisation as an indicator of the individual's performance may lack rigour and the appraiser's feedback report may consequently be subjective rather than based on objective evidence. The GP quoted in Box 2.9 reflects this fear.

Box 2.9:

'Appraisal might result in "counting beans" instead of measuring practice and performance' (GP).

Another mismatch may arise if the appraisee and the appraiser (or the primary care organisation or hospital trust that the appraiser represents) have different value systems or are at odds over what they consider to be priorities. The medical professionalism project team encapsulated the fundamental principles of what being a doctor is about – *see* Box 2.10.[5] Sometimes organisational pressures and others' priorities can make it difficult for a doctor to practise in this way.

Box 2.10:   Professional principles and responsibilities of a doctor[5]

The fundamental principles:

- dedicated to serving interest of the patient
- respect for patients' autonomy
- promote social justice in the healthcare system.

Professional responsibilities. Commitment to:

- professional competence
- patients' confidentiality
- maintaining appropriate relationships with patients
- improving quality of care
- improving access to care
- a just distribution of finite resources
- scientific knowledge
- maintaining trust
- managing conflicts of interest.

Some of the uncertainty hanging over appraisal involves the lack of control that the individual has over the relaying of reports about his or her performance to others who are in powerful positions in the health service – such as the clinical governance lead, medical director, chief executive etc. Doctors are unsure about the extent to which the appraisal will be part of 'performance management' or whether it will be mainly 'formative' and supportive, helping them to develop their practice. It is important that both parties to the appraisal should agree on the contents of any report that is to be passed on to others.

Doctors fear that appraisal could be used by the authorities to force individual doctors to adopt the organisation's priorities and values, which might be to the detriment of medical professionalism and patient care.[6] A lack of agreement between both parties to the outcome of the appraisal might result in others such as the clinical governance lead of the primary care organisation or hospital trust, being drawn into the discussion at a later date to resolve any disparities.

Box 2.11:

The costs of funding appraisals of 90 GPs in West Norfolk Primary Care Trust has been put at between £100 000 and £250 000 per year.[7]

Lack of additional resources underpinning the whole appraisal process is another source of worry and discontent. Conducting the appraisal process itself, carrying out the action in personal development plans and the subsequent changes to patient care and service delivery all have significant resource implications. The commentators in Box 2.12 realise this.

Box 2.12:

'Continuing professional development allowances and support for employing locum cover should not be used for the process of appraisal – it should be used for associated educational work preparing for/arising from PDP and appraisal' (GP).

'We mustn't put all our resources into clinical substitution to cover appraisals – we need resources to address services and educational needs too' (chair of a primary care trust in England).

Although doctors have welcomed 'protected time' to complete the appraisal paperwork and prepare for and undertake the appraisal interview, many GPs have doubts about the limited extent of GP locum time that may be provided and fear that funds for such locum cover may be drawn from patient care. Those quoted in Boxes 2.13 and 2.14 give some idea of the time spent in preparing for appraisal, even by well-organised doctors.

Box 2.13:

A consultant rheumatologist described his experience of an appraisal by an experienced chest physician. He took five days to prepare his portfolio and complete the paperwork, spending about five hours overall. His task was easier than for many of his colleagues, he said, as he was meticulous about keeping good records of his continuing professional development.

Consultants and GPs know that they will still have to catch up on their everyday work and anticipate a heavy workload on their return, even if emergency cover has been provided while they prepared for their appraisal and during the appraisal discussion itself.

Box 2.14:

'We're so busy; we don't need this – we know we're practising okay already' (practising GP).

'I reckon it took eight hours to get everything together to prepare for and do my appraisal' (GP participating in the piloting of appraisal in Wales).

An agreed action plan will be too superficial if neither the appraiser nor the appraisee are in a position to remedy underlying weaknesses in the organisational systems or reverse the inadequate resources that contributed to the individual's underperformance identified at the appraisal.

It will be difficult for a primary care organisation or hospital trust to dispel most of these fears until the appraisal process has been established for some considerable time and trust has been built up. As long as appraisal is a uniformly positive and supportive process, individual doctors should feel that the effort involved in collecting information and evidence about their work and preparing the appraisal paperwork is more than compensated for by the benefits that ensue from appraisal.

Box 2.15:

A medical director of one trust described how appraisal had become accepted in his hospital trust. 'I think the lesson for other trusts is that if you introduce things sensitively, doctors are less conservative than people think they are. You have to offer people opportunities to make constructive change.'[4]

Benefits of appraisal

Such benefits will include official recognition for the good work that doctors are doing in their everyday practice. Benefits will also relate to practical help with solving organisational difficulties. Such help might concern amending the management of staff or services, or finding new or differently targeted resources. This might mean redirecting resources at the service development needs that were identified through the appraisal process, or funding specific educational opportunities agreed in the appraisee's PDP. An ultimate outcome of the appraisal process will be the acceptance of doctors' successfully completed appraisal folders as the majority of the evidence they have to submit to obtain revalidation.

Box 2.16:   Examples of benefits emerging from consultant appraisal

In one hospital trust, a number of job plans of individual consultants have been re-negotiated, based on the evidence provided at their appraisals. 'One department achieved a new consultant appointment purely on the grounds of workload. With very few exceptions, the process has been reported as positive, has ensured that the issues around workload are understood by the organisation, and has helped individuals and departments in their annual planning cycles.'[1]

Appraisals should help medical staff feel more valued – many consultants have said they don't otherwise get praised for their work. Appraisals may make doctors more aware of the needs and aims of a hospital trust.

Box 2.17:   A consultant surgeon is won over by his appraisal[4]

Bob, a neurologist, gained a lot from his appraisal despite his initial doubts. As he was a new consultant in the plastic surgery unit, he welcomed the appraiser giving him guidance as he was working in a new area away from his previous network of support and advice.

His appraiser discussed ideas for re-organising the department and promoting its work, giving Bob the confidence to take things forward. 'He reassured me that I was doing all right. As a new consultant there are lots of things which I am a bit scared about and he gave me guidance.'

Box 2.18:   A consultant working in accident and emergency (A&E) describes his mainly positive experience of appraisal[4]

Keith focused on cardiology – which he found to be one of the more difficult parts of his work – when he took part in the voluntary appraisal scheme at the Norfolk and Norwich Trust. 'In A&E you rarely get feedback unless something has gone wrong – this gave me the opportunity to look at what had happened,' he is reported as saying. He traced patients he had seen with suspected cardiology problems and a colleague peer reviewed his treatment of them, informed by the eventual outcome. He subsequently went on a four-day course which improved his ability to interpret electrocardiograms.

The questionnaire about his interaction with other staff, which was sent to a cross-section of people he worked with, triggered lots of positive reports. He commented that 'I have a bit of a fan club out there'.

He concluded, 'I'm not half as negative as I was [about appraisal] the first time round ... it allows me to say this is what I'm good at and this is where

continued opposite

I can improve ... it has made me think about my future. It's important to think about where you want to be in five years' time. Overall, I'm very positive about appraisal.'

One drawback that he found was the huge amount of time involved, not only for him and the colleague reviewing his work, but also for his secretary and the medical records division.

NHS fears about the appraisal process

It is not only the appraisee who has fears about the appraisal process, but also the responsible primary care organisation and hospital trust. The new appraisers and those to whom the appraisers report may be anxious too. They may be uncertain about:

- how useful or cost-effective the process will be
- how appraisal will be regarded by doctors who are appraising or being appraised
- whether individual doctors will support the process or sabotage it.

For instance, doctors might seem to co-operate with preparing and submitting an appraisal folder, but in reality they may only select information about their performance that shows them in a good light and conceals their imperfections. If such behaviour were the norm, this would fuel an atmosphere of concealment rather than the open learning culture that the NHS aspires to achieve for its workforce.

There are circumstances where the relationship between the two people involved in the appraisal may create difficulties, or even undermine the whole process. If the appraisal is too 'cosy' a process, there may be collusion between the two – and this will reduce its usefulness and may even perpetuate poor practice. The appraiser may be junior to the appraisee in other areas of work. If personalities or hierarchical structures are such that the appraiser lacks confidence in relating to the more senior appraisee, the power imbalance may wreck the quality of the two-way exchange of information and discussion – as illustrated by the example of a poor appraisal in Box 2.19.

An appraisee may start off the appraisal interview itself being angry or hostile at being summoned to account for their practice – as they see it. Even an experienced appraiser may be unable to defuse the tension sufficiently in the time available, to move forward and reach a meaningful discussion with action planning. The appraiser may choose to halt the appraisal in this situation, discuss the appraisee's issues and reconvene the appraisal interview at a later date.

Box 2.19:

One appraisal of a senior doctor, undertaken by an inexperienced appraiser, started out with the quaking appraiser asking: 'How do you think we should do this?' The difficulty was that they had not exchanged paperwork prior to the day of the interview and there was no previous appraisal record to review or compare current performance. The appraiser proceeded to settle some old scores while he had the opportunity to force his senior colleague, the appraisee, to listen to a subjective review of his last year's work.

Box 2.20:

One hospital consultant has reported how difficult it is for an appraiser from outside a specialty to be able to assess the performance of a consultant from a different specialty. However, if the alternative is to appoint a work colleague as an appraiser, he or she may not have sufficient objectivity. 'For some specialties like A&E it is harder to keep a check on consultants than, say, surgery where the results of the quality of your work are obvious. In A&E it is quantity that is measured rather than quality, so consultants who have developed bad habits over the years are hard to catch out. You need to be appraised by someone from outside your specialty – if it was a colleague, you'd choose your best friend – but no-one knows about A&E except someone who works there.'

It may be difficult to collect robust evidence about a doctor's practice or performance if he or she is not co-operative. He or she may not be willing to share the results of internal clinical audits or dissect his or her part in a team effort.

Primary care organisations and hospital trusts will have fears similar to those held by individual doctors. They will be concerned that there are insufficient resources to do justice to the information and evidence about learning needs of the medical workforce and gaps in service delivery that can be deduced from pooled data from doctors' appraisals. Unbalanced or incorrectly analysed information will lead to poor decision-making.

What everyone can do to dispel fears about the appraisal process

The key will be to establish a learning culture of which appraisal is a part, so that there are resources targeted at helping to address the gaps and issues identified by regular appraisals of the entire workforce. Appraisal should be presented as a positive and motivating process with constructive outcomes.

> **Box 2.21:**
>
> The NHS will need to work hard to evolve into a 'learning organisation' with the supportive approach to all its workforce that the term conveys.
>
> One senior GP has written: 'So now everything is different. It is expected after years of bullying, harassment and bludgeoning, that we should now not only admit our dreadful mishaps in significant event monitoring to our peers, but we should also submit ourselves to probing enquiries about our performance ... [but then he goes on] ... With new supportive mechanisms in place, perhaps we can start to value each other again at whatever stage in our career we have reached and then perhaps the public will value us more, too.'[8]

Exchange the appraisal paperwork in good time

The exchanging of information in the completed appraisal paperwork between the two people involved in the appraisal should take place in plenty of time prior to the appraisal meeting – aim for three or so weeks before. This should give the appraisee time to collect additional evidence if he or she thinks that the appraiser's information is incorrect or misleading. It gives the appraisee an opportunity to reflect on the likely content and outcomes of the forthcoming appraisal discussion. Similarly, the appraiser can familiarise him or herself with the information about the appraisee's practice and can start thinking through the main issues for the appraisal discussion.

Train and support appraisers well

The choice and training of appraisers is key to the creation of a robust appraisal system that everyone can trust. The individual doctor being appraised, the primary care organisation or hospital trust, the General Medical Council or a member of the general public all need to trust the judgement and impartiality of the appraiser. An appraiser should be 'a clinician who is well respected by his or her professional peers and who can gain the confidence of those he or she will appraise. Appraisers should have the confidence of the local primary care organisation (or hospital trusts etc.)'.[6]

Qualities for which an appraiser should be able to demonstrate competence in the portfolio of evidence are given in Box 2.22.

Box 2.22: Well-trained appraisers should be competent in the following qualities.

1   Understand the healthcare context relevant to the appraisee and make realistic allowances for problems and issues that might obstruct the application of best practice.
2   Understand the potential for conflicts of interest to arise between the appraiser and the appraisee; and between the appraisee and the hospital trust or primary care organisation or the wider NHS.
3   Understand the national priorities and NHS approach to performance and how this is relevant to the appraisee's circumstances.
4   Understand and practise principles of adult education:
    • give good feedback to the appraisee, verbally and in a written report
    • guide the appraisee to identify his or her personal learning and service development needs
    • help the appraisee to set educational objectives
    • encourage an appraisee to make a relevant and realistic learning plan within his or her PDP for the coming year and beyond
    • help the appraisee to evaluate the contents of his or her PDP
    • motivate the appraisee to formulate and carry out his or her PDP
    • empower the appraisee with regard to self-improvement.
5   Understand and practise skills in interpersonal working and communication, being:
    • non-judgemental
    • generous in their praise
    • able to listen and *hear* in a positive manner
    • skilled in communicating well in a systematic way
    • able to establish a rapport with all appraisees, whatever their backgrounds
    • competent to reach consensus with the appraisee about his or her action plan, through discussion.
6   Understand and practise skills in undertaking annual appraisal.
7   Understand the structure and process of appraisal and help the appraisee to navigate through the paperwork and appraisal process as necessary.
8   Understand the standards of information and evidence expected and be able to demonstrate standards of information and evidence between an 'excellent', 'good enough' and 'unacceptable' appraisal folder.

(Adapted from Chambers.[9] These qualities are described in more depth in Chapter 10.)

Appraisers are bound to experience ongoing problems, with the appraisal process or difficult individuals, that they had not anticipated and will need support. This might be solved by networking with other appraisers, or by special help from the deaneries and their GP and clinical tutors' systems. There may be someone with a wealth of experience in each locality who is responsible for supporting appraisers and arranging further ongoing training. For instance, the appraisers may want to discuss who owns any personal notes they make during the appraisal interviews – notes that are outside of the official paperwork they pass onto the responsible organisation or trust.

Appraisers will require appropriate support in terms of financial recompense and protected time for their role in the appraisal process. Appraisers will need to be kept abreast of any amendments to the appraisal paperwork or process, or publication of new governmental directives or GMC guidance, which affect the standards or evidence required at appraisal.

Box 2.23:

'The Royal College of General Practitioners welcomes appraisal in principle ... we believe an educational structure which is supportive of GPs will boost patients' confidence and overcome the professional isolation experienced by many family doctors.'

(Professor David Haslam, Chair of Council of RCGP, February 2002)

Arrange interim reviews of progress between appraiser and appraisee

As the appraiser quoted in the example in Box 2.24 indicates, appraisal should not be regarded as a purely annual process. Depending on time and capacity, the two involved in the appraisal should meet or communicate (e.g. by phone or email) to keep a check on how the appraisee's personal development plan and other action-planning is progressing mid-year. This will take considerable organisation, especially if an appraiser is responsible for appraising many doctors, some of whom show worrying underperformance and require remedial help.

Box 2.24:

A consultant, newly trained as an appraiser, stated: 'Appraisal is not something you are going to do once a year. There should be no shocks for someone being appraised as there should have been good communication between the appraiser/appraised in the preceding year.'

NHS organisations represented by appraisers should have realistic expectations of doctors' standards of practice

There should be a close understanding, between the appraisers and the NHS primary and secondary care organisations that they are representing, about the scope of the appraisal and the standards that they are expecting doctors to reach.

Appraisers should appreciate what a competent medical practitioner does as a basis for understanding an individual's particular post. When interpreting how the individual doctor works, they should remember that:

- a generalist excludes serious disease, accepts uncertainty, explores probability and marginalises danger
- a specialist confirms serious disease, reduces uncertainty, explores possibilities and marginalises error.[10]

It is difficult to define exactly what qualities a competent doctor demonstrates. Box 2.25 describes the characteristics of a competent GP; the list may be just as applicable to doctors from other specialties.

Box 2.25:   What a competent GP does

1   Assimilates information from multiple sources rapidly.
2   Makes intuitive decisions (hypothesis testing and not protocol driven).
3   Negotiates health and social outcomes.
4   Has depth and breadth of knowledge and skills.
5   Acts independently and takes responsibility at a high professional level.
6   Handles uncertainty by means of a risk management approach.
7   Cares consistently for patients whatever their backgrounds.

(Personal communication, T Davies and M Vaughan, 2002[11])

Any concerns that a primary care organisation or hospital trust has about an individual doctor's performance should be based on evidence rather than other people's impressions or assertions. This may mean the appraiser seeking to 'triangulate' such information before the appraisal meeting – maybe gathering information from other external inspections or reviews recently carried out, about prescribing or referrals, or comparative audits etc.

Quality assurance

External quality assurance by an independent body that is not involved in the delivery of appraisal will go a long way to allaying the sort of fears described in this chapter.

Primary care organisations and hospital trusts should be monitoring the appraisals undertaken on their behalf and reviewing how appraisers perform over time with different individuals. Hopefully the monitoring will reveal benefits to justify the hopes as expressed in Boxes 2.26 and 2.27.

Box 2.26:

'I remain convinced that appraisal is a positive move, and one that will be of benefit to the NHS, doctors and, most importantly, patients.'

(Dr David Graham, Postgraduate Dean, Mersey Deanery; Chair of the Appraisal Steering Group for England, May 2002[12])

Box 2.27: Benefits of appraisals: experience over four years in a general practice

'Having been involved in GP appraisal for four years, I can say with confidence that, done well, appraisal is empowering and yields many benefits to the GP and to the practice as a whole.

'When we introduced our appraisal system at Bellevue Medical Centre, there was a reluctance to participate (particularly among the doctors!), but when the benefits became apparent, there was universal support. We found that it supported the practice's service development and helped us to plan our practice learning sessions as well as addressing individual needs. As a result of the appraisal process, one partner embarked on an MBA course using prolonged study leave and another successfully completed her MRCGP modules. The practice targeted communication skills and cardiovascular disease in its learning sessions for all staff and introduced a monthly critical event meeting.

'A big lesson for us was the realisation of the time commitment needed to make appraisal successful. We found that each appraisal took 90 minutes (we thought it would only take about 45 minutes at the most). The preparation by the GP (appraisee) took at least as long. The appraiser also prepared by talking to staff members in a confidential 360° process. Time is critical – the time spent on appraisal has meant a small reduction in the number of appointments available for patients, but in the long run we believe that the benefits for the practice and the patients outweigh the investment.'

(Professor Steve Field, Bellevue Medical Centre, 2002)

References

1 Black D (2002) Consultant appraisal – one year on: personal review. *GMC News. Supplement on Appraisal and Revalidation.* 1–4.

2 Irvine S and Jelley D (2001) *The Peer Appraisal Handbook for GPs.* Radcliffe Medical Press, Oxford.

3 King J (2002) 360° appraisal. *BMJ Careers.* **324**: s195–6.

4 Moore A (2001) Turned to good account. In: M Crail (ed.) *Leadership in the NHS.* Health Service Journal, London.

5 Medical Professionalism Project (2002) *Lancet.* **359**: 520–2.

6 Leech P (2001) *Training: annual appraisal for general practitioners.* Letter to Chief Executives of Primary Care Trusts and Primary Care Groups, Department of Health, London.

7 Bostock N (2002) PCTs struggle to find enough cash for GP appraisals. *Primary Care Report.* **24 April**: 3.

8 Archard G (2002) Reflections on the past – hopes for the future. *GMC News. Supplement on Appraisal and Revalidation.* 1–4.

9 Chambers R (2002) *A Guide to Accredited Professional Development: pathway to revalidation.* Royal College of General Practitioners, London.

10 Marinker M (1998) *General Practice and the New Contract.* In: Bevan and Marinker (eds) *Greening the White Paper.* Social Market Foundation, London.

11 Davies T and Vaughan M (2002) Welsh Council, Royal College of General Practitioners (unpublished).

12 Graham D (2002) View from the top. *Hospital Doctor.* **30 May**: 22.

3

The appraisal interview

You have two months' notice of your appraisal date. Don't panic! You have already kept your appraisal folder throughout the year (you didn't skip the previous chapter, did you?) so you are well prepared to face the music. The information you have collected will also link together with the General Medical Council's requirements for revalidation, so that you are only amassing one set of records. Look at Part 2 of this book for how you might go about making these links.

Who will be doing the appraisal?

Wherever you work, your appraiser should be someone in the same field of work as yourself, or with an understanding of your work. He or she will have volunteered (in a moment of enthusiasm) to undergo extra training to carry out appraisals. Your appraiser will need to have a good working knowledge of the environment in which you practise. He or she will also need to know about the particular variations from standard provision that you might need to make because of the type of patients, locality, practice staffing or personal disability. You can object to the choice of appraiser if there is an incompatibility between the proposed appraiser and yourself. The chief executive or medical director will usually be responsible for nominating an alternative appraiser –

Box 3.1:

Dr Hippie had left his original GP practice to join another. They were a more relaxed group of partners who all had hobbies and interests outside medicine. The doctor nominated as his appraiser was a former partner whom Dr Hippie regarded as a driven workaholic with no sense of humour. He felt that he would not get a fair evaluation from the proposed appraiser. He asked for an alternative appraiser and was allocated instead to the GP tutor from a neighbouring area. He was pleased with the choice of appraiser, who played the saxophone just as he did, so they had a lot in common.

but that's it, so don't oppose the choice too lightly for fear of getting someone worse!

Peer review

Many doctors have special interests that will not be familiar to the appraiser. If this can be identified in advance then you can plan a review of this special interest by a peer reviewer before the appraisal interview. You may have a special interest in teaching and have kept a record of your feedback documents, or have a qualification in acupuncture with evidence of updating. GPs with special interests (GPwSIs) may have further, recently acquired qualifications, or evidence of regular reviews of their skills which can be included in their appraisal folders (also called portfolios).

Sometimes this specialised aspect may only become apparent during the appraisal interview. If it is clear that a more detailed review of this specialised aspect is required, then either you or the appraiser can request an internal or external peer review.

Box 3.2:

Dr Dermis, a GP principal, had been interested in skin disorders ever since he had acne as a teenager. He had built up expertise over the years and rarely needed to refer any but the most obscure conditions to consultant colleagues. He had no formal qualifications in dermatology and tended to assume that every GP had the same level of knowledge as him. When it became apparent in his first appraisal that he was managing conditions of much greater complexity than the average GP, it was agreed that he would go and have his knowledge and skills reviewed by one of the consultant dermatologists before his appraisal report was completed.

Such a peer review is expected to take place within a month. After completion, you and the appraiser then need to meet again within another month to complete the appraisal.

The portfolio career

Many health professionals do not just hold one post. With increasing experience, an interest in a particular field may have led to a part-time post in that area. Most academics in medicine like to retain some clinical work so that they do not become out of touch with the realities of patient care. A GP with a special interest may work in secondary care as a clinical assistant or a hospital practitioner. A consultant may work in occupational medicine, do private work or take on palliative care in a hospice. Others, both GPs and consultants, may have developed their interests in education and training by working as course organisers or clinical tutors. The variations are legion. It is not yet clear how appraisal will work for this group of people and there will have to be a period of experimentation to determine how it will work in practice. There may be appraisal systems in place that affect their work in their area of special interest and that will need to be adapted in the future (e.g. deanery appraisal systems).

If a doctor's special interest is only a small part of his or her main occupation, then it may be appropriate to include it in the evidence for the appraisal. Arrange for a peer review or include evidence of competency and keeping up to date as in the previous section.

For some people there is no 'main occupation' – just several differing strands. This might mean negotiation between the appraisers appointed by different responsible bodies or the undertaking of a joint appraisal.

Box 3.3:

Dr Guide still continues his work as a hospital consultant, although he has agreed a reduction to working half-time with his hospital trust. The rest of his working week is taken up as a senior lecturer in the medical school. He has two appraisals planned – one for his academic work and one in his hospital trust. He asks his appraisers to discuss which aspects they wish to cover from the paperwork that he prepares and supplies to both. He has already drafted a PDP for both of his posts, using elements from both to eliminate overlap and demonstrate action plans in each of the two fields.

On 30 January 2001, the Secretary of State for Health presented the report of the Royal Liverpool Children's Inquiry (the Redfern Report) to the House of Commons.[1] It caused a major public outcry. One of the resulting actions was the establishment, by the Secretary of State for Education and Employment, of a review of the accountability and management arrangements between NHS trusts and universities where senior staff are employed on joint contracts. Sir Brian Follett and Michael Paulson-Ellis were asked to review the appraisal, disciplinary and reporting arrangements for joint appointments between the NHS and universities.[2] They published their report in September 2001, which is summarised in Box 3.4.

Colleges and institutions have, or will be setting down, their requirements for revalidation. This will enable individuals who have attained a qualification in, for example, occupational medicine, family planning or sports medicine to demonstrate that they have met the requirements for revalidation. This

Box 3.4: Appraisal for doctors and dentists with academic and clinical duties: an introduction to the Follett Report

The authors of the Follett Report stated that the key principle for NHS and university organisations involved in medical education and research should be 'joint working to integrate separate responsibilities'. They felt that university and NHS partnerships responsible for medical education and research should establish joint strategic planning bodies, with joint subsidiary bodies responsible for staff management policies and procedures for staff with academic and clinical duties.

They suggested that substantive and honorary contracts for senior NHS and university staff posts with academic and clinical duties should be explicit about separate lines of responsibility, reporting arrangements and staff management procedures, and should be consistent, cross-referenced and issued as a single package. This also meant that any substantive university contract and honorary NHS contract for clinical academics should be interdependent. They recognised that medical education was no longer restricted to partnerships between a university and one or more teaching hospitals. It referred, therefore, to NHS bodies rather than hospitals or trusts, reflecting that academic general practice in particular was playing an increasingly important part in medical education.

The authors placed appraisal at the heart of their report. They said that they believed that regular annual appraisal had the capacity to lead to considerable change and improvement. They concluded that universities and NHS bodies should work closely together to develop a jointly agreed annual appraisal and performance review process based on that for NHS consultants, to meet the needs of both partners. They said that the process should:

- involve a decision on whether single or joint appraisal is appropriate for every senior NHS and university staff member with academic and clinical duties
- ensure joint appraisal for clinical academics holding honorary consultant contracts and for NHS staff undertaking substantial roles in universities
- define joint appraisal as two appraisers, one from the university and one from the NHS, working with one appraisee on a single occasion
- require a structured input from the other partner where a single appraiser acts
- be based on a single set of documents and
- start with a joint induction for those who will be jointly appraised.

Building on the appraisal process, they also felt that universities and NHS bodies should jointly prepare a formal agreement on the procedures for the management of poor performance to be followed for senior NHS and university staff members with academic and clinical duties.

A joint steering group was established to implement their recommendations, facilitated jointly by the Department for Education and Skills and the Department of Health, with the intention of appraisal for clinical academics being introduced from April 2002. In August 2002, the Department of Health's

continued opposite

annual appraisal scheme for clinical academic consultants was finally launched. It built upon the Follett recommendations and grounded them in the principles of the general appraisal scheme for consultants. The guidance is available on the DoH website, www.doh.gov.uk/nhsexec/consultantappraisal.

What this means for you
In your working environment, therefore, even if you spend the majority of time as an academic in the university setting, this affects you. It means that if you are an associate dean, clinical tutor, GP tutor or course organiser, you may require a joint appraisal. There may also be consequences if you are an educational supervisor or GP trainer because your appraisal should cover your educational activities even if you are to have a single NHS appraisal. You must seek to clarify what is expected of you and ensure that your appraisal follows the DoH and Follett recommendations.

Preparation is the key. It will take a lot of time! The time taken will be worth it! The range of topics to be covered in your appraisal will be wide, since on the NHS side appraisal must cover your clinical work, while on the university side it covers teaching and research, with both clinical and academic appraisals being concerned with personal and career development and any other personal issues. You must be explicit about the varying objectives required by the NHS and academic institution or deanery, although it is best that they should be combined in a single set of documentation. Careful and comprehensive record-keeping will be necessary to ensure that the material can be used as the basis for revalidation and that the process can be audited.

Your academic institution should be ready to implement the Follett recommendations; check! Ask to see the documentation and check that there is alignment of the information requirements in the appraisal process with the developing GMC criteria for the revalidation of doctors engaged in teaching and research. If there is a problem then discuss it with your medical director or chair of the professional executive committee (PEC) and with the appropriate person in the university or deanery. If there is any doubt then involve the British Medical Association (BMA) in the discussions.

Finally, be reassured. The Follett recommendations are designed to support academic staff and to protect patients; they are not designed to be punitive – they should be formative and supportive.

evidence can be included in their appraisal portfolio and should be acceptable to the appraiser even if he or she has no knowledge or skills in that field.

Some people may find that the work that they do is very fragmented and that they have to collate the evidence required in as broad a way as possible.

If most or all of the work that you do is self-employed – such as freelance writing or broadcasting – together with a small amount of locum work in general practice or as an independent doctor, it is not easy to see how this will be appraised and by whom. You may need to collect as much information and feedback as you can and show that you reflect and act on the conclusions.

Box 3.5:

Dr Busker works in many different roles. She acts as a medical adviser to a charity involved with children with handicaps and works part-time as a community paediatrician. Each week she does a community family-planning clinic and one session in a genitourinary clinic. She decides that her main interest is paediatrics and asks to be appraised in that setting. She collects evidence of her learning and performance and asks for evaluation from colleagues and patients in her other roles to put into her appraisal folder. She decides with her appraiser that some of her development plan will be generic to all her work, and some each year will apply to specific areas, to include some of the other aspects of her professional work.

There are some suggestions on how you might collect relevant evidence if you are a non-principal in general practice on the National Association of Non-Principals' website (*see* Appendix 1) and these might be adapted for use by other self-employed professionals. The medical colleges and faculties, as well as other organisations such as the British Association of Medical Managers (BAMM), are considering how the principles of good medical practice apply to non-clinical work or to medical specialties.

In the training grades, specialist registrars are catered for by their record of in-training assessment (RITA) and postgraduate deans are working to introduce RITAs and appraisal for the other grades while ensuring that there are cross-linkages to the GMC's revalidation plans.

Doctors who take a career break can be supported back into practice by the Flexible Careers Scheme (FCS) in England.[3] The scheme has been developed to enable doctors to satisfy practice criteria for appraisal and revalidation so that they can demonstrate their fitness to practise. Each doctor on the scheme will meet regularly with a clinical and educational supervisor who is also their appraiser. Locum doctors registered with the NHS Professionals organisation will also receive support and advice about appraisal and revalidation.[3]

Information on appraisal for individuals like these who do not fit into the regular appraisal pattern is available on the appraisal information website (*see* Appendix 1).

Who should be present?

In many appraisals there will be just an appraiser and an appraisee. This will make it easier to have an intimate chat. However, sometimes more people will be present. For consultants who hold academic positions there is likely to be their clinical 'line manager' (clinical director or deputy) and their academic line manager (head of academic department). For NHS consultants who hold posts in more than one hospital there might be a representative from that hospital present. The process could easily become unwieldy. The neurosciences directorate at the North Staffordshire Hospital have opted to have someone from human resources (HR) present as well as the clinical director and the appraisee. They used this system in 2001 and it worked well. The HR member took notes, so that both the appraisee and the appraiser could concentrate on the discussion. In addition, a skilled HR officer can rescue discussions when they go awry and keep the appraisee focused on the task of appraisal rather than 'belly-aching' about the NHS in general. The HR member can intervene if the appraisal strays into areas where it is inappropriate for an appraiser to go: for example, personal matters that have no bearing on job performance.

Box 3.6:   Advantages of a member of the human resources department being present at the appraisal

- Keeps notes.
- Rescues appraisals which are going awry.
- Keeps the participants focused on appraisal.
- Reminds the participants that this is a forum process.
- Keeps the appraiser in line.

Your own preparation for the appraisal interview

Successful appraisal depends on both the appraiser and appraisee giving considerable thought to their contributions beforehand. This is not an examination, but an exploration of what you do, how well you can do it and what stops you doing things better. There will be areas where you know you are doing well – and others where you know that you, or the set-up at your workplace or in your area, are deficient.

Box 3.7:

The Department of Health for England suggests that the appraisal process would be greatly helped if both the appraiser and hospital consultant being appraised thought through the following questions before the appraisal interview.

- How good a consultant am I?
- How well do I perform?
- How up to date am I?
- How well do I work in a team?
- What resources and support do I need?
- How well am I meeting my service objectives?
- What are my development needs?

(www.revalidationuk.info[4])

Think about the barriers to better practice so that you and the appraiser can consider them together. You may want to do a little investigation of specific areas where gaps in your recording are obvious. You may want to ask other people how they do things that you would like to do or provide, so that you already have a framework for your personal development plan. The more you know about what you want to do, the more likely you are to obtain support and encouragement from your appraiser.

You should agree the time and date of the appraisal interview well in advance and make an adequate provision of time. You will need some time immediately beforehand so that you are not rushing from a surgery, clinic or visit to attend the appraisal. Think about rescheduling that day altogether so that immediately before the interview you can be catching up with paper-work, or some other activity that is controlled by you, rather than working flat out in response to the demands of others. Similarly, rearrange the appraisal or your work pattern if you are due to have the appraisal on the day after being on call during the previous night, or after travelling back from abroad across time zones.

Arrange to delegate any work during that time and ensure that you have the time protected from interruptions and distractions. There should be other people available to deal with any crisis even if someone collapses in the corridor or the car park, just as they would if you were not there. Make sure that the timing of the appraisal is convenient and sensible. It is no good trying to have a rational discussion with someone if you are anxiously awaiting news about a relative's illness or your children's examination results. You need to be able to give the appraisal interview your undivided attention at the time.

Where do you hold the appraisal?

Think about the venue. You know about the importance of the room layout for good consultation skills – so apply those skills to the room in which the appraisal will be conducted. The choice of room is important; you should select a quiet room at the right temperature. Avoid busy public rooms such as common rooms, pubs, bars or restaurants – you cannot do justice to the appraisal if others can overhear or if there are interruptions by others seeking food and drink. On the other hand, you might want to lay on some coffee, tea or soft drinks. Non-alcoholic refreshments can be useful ice-breakers and a judicious manoeuvre with a coffee cup can give you time to think.

It is absolutely essential that you are not interrupted – whether by the phone or by people entering the room. Ensure that everyone knows the room is in use, automatically bar telephone calls or remove the phone and put a large, bright notice on the door.

If your consulting room or office is the only room free, then decide who is going to sit where. Both of you will need to write things down, so arrange the chairs next to a desk. You may feel subconsciously resentful, however, if the appraiser sits in *your* chair, and uncomfortable at the difference in roles if he or she sits in the chair normally used by the patient. You might want to rearrange the room so that you sit side-by-side with the table cleared. If your desk is normally covered in papers, you could bring in another small table so that there is somewhere for all those forms to rest while you discuss them.

If the appraisal is taking place at an unfamiliar location, look at the room in advance to assess its suitability. Does it need rearranging or does it require another table? Many office environments have one chair behind the table and another facing it – remember your consultation skills and move the chairs to be at least at right angles to each other or, preferably, more like 45°. Appraisal is a conversation, not an interrogation. While comfortable chairs are a good idea, sitting in low armchairs may make note-taking difficult. Arrange the chairs so that neither of you has to look at the other silhouetted against a light from a window or lamp. It is helpful to have the chairs at equal height, otherwise anyone sitting in the lower of two chairs of unequal height will feel at a disadvantage.

What do you do in the appraisal interview?

Like all meetings between two (almost) equals, it starts with pleasantries to set both of you at ease. Your appraiser may be new to appraisal and be feeling just as anxious about the whole business as you are.

You should already know how much time has been set aside for the actual interview. This should be between an hour and an hour-and-a-half. Anything less will not be adequate to do justice to the process and the process will feel rushed, adding to the stress of the event. If the interview is too long, the focus is lost and your interchange may degenerate into conversation and anecdote.

Next, set the agenda between you. Set out what you would like to discuss – you will, of course, have jotted it down beforehand. Then make a note of what points the appraiser wants to raise. If either of you is unable to set out a plan for the meeting, then the other will tend to follow his or her own ideas. A mutually agreed plan allows time to be allocated fairly for both of you to bring forward those things that seem most important.

It should be your turn first as the appraisee. Celebrate (briefly – don't get too boastful!) your achievements and things you do well. Move on to what you would like to develop and improve. Then bring up the difficulties and barriers to the changes needed. If the appraiser wants to discuss the same topic, then don't be rigid about whose turn it is. It is better to finish one subject before starting another. Be conscious of the time and keep to the subjects that are important.

Avoid discussing the deficiencies of other people. You might acknowledge that these may play some part in the barriers that prevent certain actions on your part. However, it is a waste of valuable discussion time to spend it bewailing the poor training and skills of your staff or how much more difficult the patients that you see are than those of other colleagues. Provide facts about the problems if you have them and consider those deficiencies as challenges. Then you can ask for advice and help in overcoming them, just as you will be challenging the restraints of insufficient funds or the restrictions imposed by the lack of space in your building.

It may be that your appraiser does not see some of your achievements in quite the same light as yourself. He or she may challenge you or compare your performance with others. Be prepared to defend or explain your actions if you are sure of your ground and have the evidence to support what you have done.

Box 3.8:

Dr Hart was very pleased with the way he had built up the cardiac assessment team in his general practice. His prescriptions for statins and ACE inhibitors had escalated wildly, but he was very satisfied at the advice and management that patients who required secondary prevention were receiving. The appraiser pointed out how this had affected his prescribing figures and that he was way outside his prescribing budget. Dr Hart made a vigorous defence of his actions with evidence from the National Service Framework for Coronary Heart Disease.

Alternatively, you may be too self-critical of your performance in some areas. The appraiser may be able to point out that you are doing better than many other doctors in your field or that you have particular difficulties that hamper your efforts.

Box 3.9:

Dr Sweet was apologetic about the low level of recording for diabetes in her practice. She had been working hard to try to screen patients as she knew that she should have a far higher number. Many of her patients were of Asian origin, but had only recently arrived in Britain. They were reluctant to attend for screening, had difficulties with the language and avoided her male partner. They did not regard the practice nurse highly either!

About half the length of the interview should be taken up with looking at what has already been achieved – what is already good and might be even better. The remaining half of the interview should concentrate on the future. Your own plans and the ideas of the appraiser can come together to plan for both short-term and long-term development. These need to be realistic and achievable. Your expectations of what you can achieve in your action plan in the timescale may be too ambitious – a common failing of all doctors. Your appraiser can help you to focus on the part of your plan that is more achievable within a reasonable timescale, or suggest some interim targets so that you can measure where you are by the following year.

Box 3.10:

Dr Datum wanted to become 'paperless' in his surgery by the end of the next year. He was encouraged to aim at harmonising the coding of entries by all partners and staff by the end of the first year, before progressing to the next stage of computerisation of all practice record-keeping.

Occasionally there may be criticisms of your work by the appraiser that you were not expecting. These should be factual and should result from comparing the paperwork that you have provided with that of the standards in your area.

Box 3.11:

Dr Putty was annoyed when his appraiser pointed out that his referral rates for mole removal were the highest in the area. He told the appraiser that he had faced a complaint a couple of years ago over his alleged late referral for a mole that turned out to be a malignant melanoma. Now he referred everyone who asked his opinion about a mole to a dermatologist. He was encouraged to look at ways he could learn more about melanomas and regain his confidence in his diagnostic skills.

Most of the time there will not be any surprises. You and your appraiser will be in agreement about the standards that you are achieving. If there are differences of opinion then a consensus can usually be reached between you regarding what action should be taken.

The only person who can fail an appraisal is the appraiser. The examples given in Box 3.12 demonstrate the following:

- The appraiser does not need specialist knowledge of the clinical area, but has to be taught and have an aptitude for appraising!
- When an appraisal runs well, there is a bond of trust between appraiser and appraisee.
- The appraisee should feel confident enough to talk about his or her dreams and aspirations.
- The appraisee comes out of a good appraisal better motivated than when he/she went in.

Box 3.12: A tale of two appraisals	
I had spent half a day on appraisal training, so I thought I knew what was going to happen. Unfortunately my professor and the reader had been too busy to go to training. The whole thing went badly. They kept going on about getting publications and why was I not getting more papers out or applying for grants. I felt uncomfortable throughout. I was glad when it was over. It was just like being back at school! They offered me no help and I just felt it was a chastisement session.	I decided I wanted to have an appraisal as I knew that appraisals were coming. I also felt that I spent so much time doing things I did not have the chance to reflect where my life was going. I chose someone in the HR department to do the appraisal. I hardly knew her, but that made it easier somehow. She went through my professional life in a structured and detailed fashion and looked at my aspirations and the difficulties I was encountering. I opened up to her more than I have to anyone in my professional life before. At the end of the one-and-a-half hours I thought what a privilege it had been for someone to spend such a lot of time talking about me! I came out of the whole process feeling better about myself and remotivated to tackle some areas I had put on the back burner.

The paperwork from the appraisal interview

You will probably find it useful to keep notes on the various issues as they are discussed. Then you and the appraiser can come to a joint decision about what goes in the action plan. These notes should be confidential to you and the appraiser, but will inform your personal development plan (*see* Chapter 4 and Appendix 3) and the written overview of the appraisal.

The written overview of the appraisal should include:

- a concise account of what has been achieved in the last year
- the objectives for the action plan for the next year
- the essential elements for writing your personal development plan
- any action required by your trust to meet local needs or those in the wider community.

You will need to agree a standard summary with your appraiser as recommended by the GMC, so that this can eventually be included in your revalidation folder.

Finally, both you and your appraiser need to sign to say that you agree that the appraisal has been carried out correctly.

Both of you should keep copies of all these documents. In addition, copies of the appraisal summary, signed by both of you, are sent to the chief executive and to the clinical governance lead or senior clinical lead of your primary care organisation or hospital trust. These documents are *confidential* and *must* be held securely. Access and use must comply with the Data Protection Act.

You and the appraiser should arrange a review at least once during the course of the next year to discuss the progress of your action plan. This could be done via a telephone call, or as part of ongoing educational support.

What happens if there are serious problems?

It would be unusual for serious problems with your own performance to become apparent for the first time during an appraisal interview. The appraisal is intended to be part of an ongoing formative process.

It is possible, but very unlikely, that an appraiser may have serious concerns about the safety of patients cared for by an appraisee after undertaking the appraisal. He or she will be especially worried about an appraisee who is underperforming in some significant way(s) and appears to have no insight into these weaknesses and no plans to improve. The appraiser and appraisee should recognise that as registered medical practitioners, whether consultants or GPs, they must protect patients when they believe that a colleague's health, conduct or performance is a threat to patients. This is clearly laid out in the Department of Health and the GMC's joint guidance on appraisal on their website www.revalidationuk.info. Therefore, if as a result of the appraisal process the appraiser believes that the activities of the appraisee are such as to put patients at risk, then the appraisal process should be stopped and action taken. The GMC is clear that nothing in the operation of the appraisal process can override the basic professional obligation to protect patients.

If the appraiser is concerned, he or she should confer with senior colleagues in the primary care organisation or hospital trust regarding the appropriate action to take and discuss the situation with the medical director, GP chair of the professional executive committee (PEC) of the primary care organisation (or equivalent across the UK) or chief executive. It may be appropriate for the GMC to be notified. There should be local procedures to deal with a doctor's suspected or proven underperformance, and the appraiser can hand the matter over to those responsible. Such suspected underperformance is usually managed by correlating information from all relevant sources and further investigating the doctor's practice. The appraiser should be well aware of the duties of confidentiality to patients and should take care not to breach confidentiality or the regulations of the Data Protection Act when preparing evidence about a doctor's underperformance.

If resolution cannot be achieved or if there is disagreement, then the problem may be referred to the National Clinical Assessment Authority in England. Nothing in the appraisal process can take precedence over a doctor's professional obligation to protect patients.

What happens to the appraisal reports?

The chief executive has ultimate responsibility for appraisal, but it is the senior clinician or clinical governance lead who co-ordinates the design, implementation and conduct of appraisals. They must ensure that there are:

- arrangements for identifying, appointing and training appraisers
- processes to respond to concerns from individual doctors about the appraisal process or outcome
- actions to support the educational and developmental needs of the doctors identified by the appraisal, and to make the changes required by the service developments identified and agreed in the appraisal
- adequate financial provision to support the appraisal process such as a funded policy on locum cover.

For both hospital and general practice appraisals, it is only the forms summarising the appraisal that are sent to the chief executive, senior clinician or clinical governance lead. The senior clinician or clinical governance lead will collate the appraisals carried out throughout the year and will prepare a report on the appraisal outcomes for the chief executive. This report must not refer in any identifiable way to the individuals appraised but must be anonymised as it will be presented to the board of the primary care organisation or hospital trust. As well as being a general report on the appraisal process, this report will highlight training and development needs, and also organisational or service needs, so that the board can take action.

If you are unhappy with the appraisal process or outcome, you should put your concerns in writing to the senior clinician or clinical governance lead and the chief executive of your primary care organisation or hospital trust.

References

1 Secretary of State for Health (2001) *The Royal Liverpool Children's Inquiry. Report and summary and recommendations* (The Redfern Report). HMSO, London.

2 Follett B and Paulson-Ellis M (2001) *A Review of the Appraisal, Disciplinary and Reporting Arrangements for Senior NHS and University Staff with Academic and Clinical Duties.* Department of Education and Skills, London.

3 Department of Health (2001) *Improving Working Lives for Doctors.* Department of Health, London.

4 General Medical Council/Department of Health *Appraisal Guidance for Consultants Working in the NHS.* www.revalidationuk.info (accessed June 2002).

4

What happens after the appraisal interview?

To maximise the benefits of the effort put into the appraisal system, you should act on what you have learnt about your own practice from formally reviewing your performance. The basis for the action consists of objectives you drew up yourself for your personal development plan, any additional objectives that you agreed with your appraiser in the course of your appraisal discussion, and others derived from the appraiser's feedback report. *See* Appendix 3 for an example of a template for a personal development plan. Use the format in the appraisal paperwork (pages 190 and 194–5) or our more detailed version (pages 197–200).

The action might include:

- undertaking planned exercises to identify your particular learning needs or problems with the services or care you deliver
- following the timetabled learning plan you have drawn up in one or more specific topics in ways that suit your learning needs
- evaluating the progress you have made with learning about your chosen topic areas and any subsequent changes in your practice, behaviour or attitudes
- your role and responsibilities in teamwork in the areas upon which you are focusing.

Finalising your personal development action plan

Your appraisal should have concluded with an agreed action plan which you and your appraiser are committed to implementing. This will have your revised personal development plan at its core. If you have kept on top of your personal development plan over the last year, you will already have justified what you plan to learn as a priority in the coming twelve months. Thus, there should be few changes, unless your own personal priorities are not synchronised with those of your primary care organisation or hospital trust.

Finding resources to carry out your personal development plan

Even the most conscientious and driven doctor will not meet his or her objectives without the support of the hospital trust or primary care organisation. Support means resources, both in terms of money and the freedom to take time away from the ward, clinic, theatre or consulting room. Improving performance of individuals requires commitment from the organisation and the individual; the appraisal interview can be quite demoralising if that support is not transparent and resources are inaccessible.

It is important, therefore, that at the appraisal interview, the appraiser has anticipated the need for resources and, if possible, is in a position to support you. After your appraisal interview, attempt to secure the resources that you need to progress your PDP. It is relatively easier to pledge to carry out action and learning when you are sitting comfortably away from the fray of clinical practice than when you are back to the reality of having little spare time and limited funds for course fees or locum cover.

Identifying resources for your PDP will include finding:

- time
- appropriate courses or sources of learning about your prioritised areas
- fees to undertake courses or pay for the help of an expert
- help from colleagues to allow you to apply your learning in practice.

Identifying sufficient time will include attendance at a meeting, a course or even a secondment. Private study should also figure prominently in achieving your objectives. Set aside time to reflect after each learning event. Consider how to apply what you have learnt, as an individual or with your team, in your everyday practice. Additional time may be required to meet up with your appraiser or GP/clinical tutor again for an interim review of your revised PDP.

Opportunities for learning might be local or distant, necessitating travel and overnight expenses. You should think creatively about how best to learn what you need to know. It may not be seeking out an appropriate course but choosing to shadow someone else or arranging a tutorial from an expert.

You may need to find the money for fees to undertake courses or even pay for the help of an expert mentor or external consultant. These might include the fees for registering for a higher degree or professional quality award. You may require extra funds for an external review of your services or care, or assessment of your application for a national recognition of quality award, for example, the 'Investors in People' award. The Department of Health's *Advance Letter [(MD) 6/00]* described the agreement on appraisal for NHS consultants in England: 'To be successful, the appraisal scheme must be introduced with an appropriate level of support for appraisers and appraisees. Adequate time should be allocated for preparation.'

Funding may also be needed to cover staff time/skills or other costs such as equipment. These should be relevant to changes in service delivery that are either essential or desirable, if you are to apply what you will have gained from your personal development activities. They might include staff time to carry out preliminary work establishing baselines to enable changes to be evaluated, for obtaining patients' or staff's views and feedback, or for information technology support, etc. You may need to buy resources to underpin your and your colleagues' learning activities and everyday practice. The resources might include access to updated computers to enable systematic clinical audit, electronic databases to ease the adoption of evidence in practice, a locally based library service, etc. Do not forget to include the future costs of colleagues and staff who cover service work that you stop doing once you have attained the new skills you plan to gain.

You will probably need the help of colleagues in putting your newly gained skills into practice. This might mean including them in applying new guidelines, protocols or procedures that are an integral part of your planned improvements. You may need to organise a local meeting of hospital consultants and general practitioners to agree new ways of working together, revising, printing and disseminating new guideline folders, etc.

There will be many requirements for additional resources emerging from your PDP if it is to be carried out in a meaningful way and change your practice.

The responsibility for identifying some of these resources will rest with your hospital trust or primary care organisation – for example, additional library or IT resources. Others will fall upon your team in the practice or hospital department as, for instance, you revise the skill mix in the way you deliver services to patients. Some will fall upon you – such as time for reflection and updating of your PDP.

Reaching a compromise about what you could and will learn and apply from your PDP

Much of the learning and action arising from your PDP will be a matter of compromise between what your aspirations are and the reality of limited time and resources. Reaching a compromise will be a matter of judging what is possible in your everyday work, and the constraints such as those arising from your team or colleagues, your family and personal situation etc.

The costs of learning more about your priority areas in an 'ideal' way may be too high, and you may have to settle for an 'acceptable' method of learning. For instance, ideally you might want to attend a week-long course which has national recognition, but is sited a long way from your home. Instead, you opt for a local two-day course that costs less and takes up less time. As your time and funds may be severely limited, you will have to think about other compromises you need to make.

Reach a fair balance between the proportion of time and funds you spend on addressing your weaknesses and that spent on building on your strengths in refining or advancing your skills. Match the extent of effort you put into the learning that benefits the organisation or practice in which you work and the personal advantages to you from increasing your qualifications and skills, enabling you to earn more money or transfer to another post.

Conflicting priorities might concern tensions between your personal aspirations and those of colleagues in your workplace. For instance, in a hospital team, another consultant colleague may already be an expert in the area that you would dearly like to develop or specialise in, or in general practice, a GP partner may already lead on a clinical or management area that fascinates you too.

You may have to compromise in the extent to which you disseminate what you have learnt from your PDP to other colleagues in your practice or department or, further afield, across your hospital trust, primary care organisation or the wider NHS. There are limits to your time and energy in how much dissemination the primary care organisation or hospital trust can expect you to achieve.

Similarly, there may be conflicting priorities between the perspectives of your appraiser, who is employed by the primary care organisation or hospital trust and so is ostensibly representing its interests, and those of the wider NHS. For instance, your patient population may suffer from a particular health problem that you want to learn more about but which does not match with nationally set clinical priorities.

Your appraiser should be a medical colleague who is 'fully acquainted with relevant areas of expertise and knowledge' as far as your work is concerned. However, it may not have been possible to find such a colleague if you are working in an unusual specialty or advanced area, and the appraiser might not appreciate issues that affect how you prioritise or undertake activities in your PDP.

Conflict may arise from two or more components of your regular work programme and everyday responsibilities. For instance, you may have two or more contracts in different specialty areas, such as medical practice and academic work. Each of these specialties will require a different focus on learning, and some topics may be more urgent than others. There is potential for conflict around priorities, funding to undertake learning and time away from work in pursuit of the parts of the PDP that are not relevant to one post but are to the other.

Lastly, you will have to develop a method to balance your planned priorities against those new ones that crop up at work in the subsequent twelve months and swamp your previous intentions. You will need to anticipate whether your appraiser next year will accept that you were justified in allowing the new priorities to entirely overturn those that you had previously agreed were priorities for your current PDP. You can always sound out the appraiser on this at any interim review.

Feeding into the training plan

Appraisal will identify educational needs of individuals, practices, departments and hospitals. If appraisal works well, it should feed into educational planning and allow the resources to be directed to the areas of need. If, for example, ten doctors within a primary care organisation or a hospital identified communication skills training as one of their developmental needs, then rather than sending them individually on expensive courses it may be more cost-effective and supportive for the individuals to bring in a trainer and run in-house training.

Decide how you will evaluate your PDP before you start

First, you should consider what sort of outcomes you are aiming for from your appraisal and personal development plan. Then these outcomes should be matched by appropriate methods that evaluate the extent to which you will have achieved your plans.

You might evaluate whether:

- you created a reasonable amount of protected time for learning
- the contents of your PDP were relevant to your needs
- you have learnt what you set out to do
- you identified your particular learning needs or problems with the services or care you deliver appropriately
- you adopted a meaningful approach to reflective learning
- you followed the timetabled learning plan you drew up twelve months ago
- you made changes to the care of patients and improvements in health or social outcomes for patients

- you fulfilled your role and responsibilities in teamwork in the areas you focused on.

The methods you might use to evaluate your everyday work and the achievements from your personal development plan will probably be similar to those you used to identify your learning needs and capture baseline information about your performance. You may simply repeat that method as you complete your PDP. For instance, you might run a clinical audit before and after you have learnt about the topic and applied your learning in practice. You could look at any aspects of the structure, process and outcome of a service or project to see if you have achieved what you expected to learn or apply.

You could build your evaluation on any or all of the six aspects of the NHS performance assessment framework: health improvement, fair access, effective delivery, efficiency, patient–carer experience, health outcomes.[1]

You might agree milestones or goals in terms of knowledge and skills or service implementation at any stage of your personal development plan, or adopt others such as those set out in national guidance – for example, on coronary heart disease or cancer services.

You could evaluate your technical competence or your knowledge, skills and the effectiveness of the treatments you provide. You could look at the aspects of care that are highly valued by patients such as your communication skills, including your ability to explore patients' needs, listen, explain, give information and involve them in decision-making.

There is no one right way to evaluate your work – just choose a method that suits your purpose.[2,3]

Serious concerns arising from the appraisal

An appraiser would not be expected to be the main person to lead on providing developmental and educational support to an appraisee. If an appraisee requires substantial support after the appraisal discussion to put together or action any part of the PDP, that is likely to be derived from a GP or clinical tutor, a college tutor or from the local deanery's educational team.

There should be clear local procedures, both in the hospital and primary care settings, to address any concerns from the individual doctors about the process, outcome or use of information. A system of mediation involving the medical director or clinical governance lead would be appropriate, with the ultimate appeal, in exceptional circumstances, to a board convened by the chief executive for disputes that cannot be resolved.

References

1 Department of Health (2001) *NHS Performance Indicators: a consultation.* Department of Health, London.

2 Wakley G, Chambers R and Field S (2000) *Continuing Professional Development in Primary Care: making it happen.* Radcliffe Medical Press, Oxford.

3 Chambers R (2002) *A Guide to Accredited Professional Development: pathway to revalidation.* Royal College of General Practitioners, London.

5

Overcoming barriers to making the most of appraisal

You have drawn up your action plan within your personal development plan (PDP) – so now what? You will probably find yourself delaying, putting off starting, and finding excuses why you cannot begin just yet. It is difficult to contemplate change, acquire new knowledge or skills and alter what you do.

Look at the flow chart in Figure 5.1 showing how people react to change.

We start off by being taken by surprise about a change even if we anticipated it. You will feel more comfortable if the action plan that you have drawn up is based on what you want to do. You will be less happy with modifications to your working practice if the changes are forced upon you by variations in the services you provide or the requirements of your job. There is still a shock element when a change first occurs and for a while we are not quite sure what has happened. We move from that shock to pretending it is not going to happen, or that it will do so magically without any input from ourselves. For example, we all know some doctors who are still denying that revalidation will happen and will go away if they ignore it. When we hear about 'improving

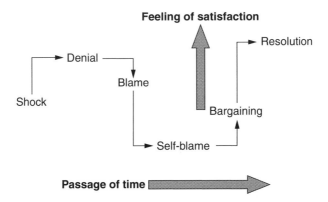

Figure 5.1: Reacting to change.

quality' or 'consulting the public', some people say, 'Oh no, there will be something else in place by the time I need to do it, so I won't bother with it now.'

After the denial phase in the change process, we move on to find somebody else to blame for what has happened – and we tend to blame the messengers. For example, you may feel antagonism or anger towards your appraiser, or the primary care organisation/hospital trust, for setting standards or objectives – as though somehow it is their fault that this has to happen.

After the stage of blaming others comes self-blame. We say, 'What if I'm not good enough?' or 'What if I can't do it in the time?' and express our worries and insecurities. If these are serious and hold up the progress of the change through to resolution, you may need to seek some help from your tutor, mentor or other source.

Then we move on to the bargaining stage. People say, 'Well, if I show I can do it this way, perhaps I can get some help from the trust' or 'If I do this part this year, perhaps next year I can get some funding to do that the following year.' In this way, we try to balance things up.

When introducing change we have to aim to *do things in a different way* rather than just *doing more things* and piling activities on top of each other. That is part of the bargaining – if we do it this way we are going to have more time to do that as well. Eventually we arrive at the resolution phase where we have accepted the change.

We pass through these different stages of change according to how we are as people. We all know the people who are always enthusiastic for change and who rush through these processes. These are the 'early adopters' who often spend little time thinking about the consequences of their actions and, as a result, have to make other modifications soon afterwards, sometimes even reverting to the previous position. Others, 'laggards', drag their feet and wait until everyone else has made the necessary alterations, often missing out on the advantages such as pump priming funding. The middle way allows enough time for reflection, as well as taking advantage of innovations. We often move to different phases of that change cycle depending on who we are talking to and what we perceive to be the threats around us.

What affects how quickly we move through the flow chart of change?

When change is imposed on us, we are very much resistant, so we move more slowly. If the effects of the change are serious, our feelings about the change will be stronger. If at the end of the action plan we think we are going to lose our job, role or status, we can be very much more upset by a change.

Box 5.1:

Dr Otis has been the expert on managing discharging ears. He has agreed to spend time during the next twelve months developing a nurse-led service. The nurses will gradually take over the management from him. He feels reluctant to start despite knowing that the nurses can become as skilled as he is. He is mollified by 'bargaining' that, once the nurses are competent, he can set up a clinic for ear problems. He has obtained agreement from the primary care trust to fund this clinic to provide a resource for less complicated problems that do not require the expertise of secondary care.

Box 5.2:

Consultant dermatologist Dr Spot identified a need to support his local general practices, and help reduce waiting times, in his PDP at his appraisal. He agreed to work with his nurses and with local GPs and their nurses to develop new guidelines for referral. He proposed a new service where local GPs emailed digital photos of patients' rashes and spots as well as their clinical histories, so that advice could be given more quickly without the need for patients to consult him at the hospital. The hospital committed resources for a pilot project which included training, digital cameras and freeing up nursing time to manage the project.

How do you learn to cope with change?

First, remind yourself that you were actually dissatisfied with how things were and drew up an action plan to alter and improve the situation. If you and your appraiser had been satisfied with the situation at your appraisal then you might have concluded: 'If it ain't broke, don't fix it.'

Next, you need to have a clear idea of where you are going. When you audit what you do, or reflect on significant events, you are constantly monitoring your level of satisfaction. You have to decide which of those mountains over there you are actually going to climb. The terrain across which you have to travel is different if you are heading for this mountain on the right than if you are travelling towards the mountain on the left. You need clear objectives – and you should have drawn these up in your personal development plan (*see* Chapter 4 and Appendix 3).[1]

You need to map out how you are going to reach that target – that mountain over there. You have to find your way in staged steps and read signposts on the way to actually getting there. You need a clear action plan of how to reach your objectives.[2] The following considerations will help you reach your mountain:

- Have realistic timescales. If they are unrealistic, you will not want to start and you will become disillusioned and unmotivated.

Box 5.3:

Dr Clutter, a paediatrician, had been asked to write a protocol for managing diarrhoea in infants and children. He was told it had to be in place in three months' time. At his appraisal he shared his frustration about this management decision and was helped to draw up a more reasonable timescale. It was agreed that he could not write workable protocols in three months. He drew up a schedule for the consultations that would be required, the revisions that would then be done, and a plan for involving all the relevant people necessary for the implementation of the protocol.

- Use clear communication. People need to know what is going on. You need to set up lines of communication to all the people who are going to be affected right at the outset. You need to be able to hear what they are saying as well so that as soon as rumours spring up, you can feed back the correct information. If you deal with those quickly then you can pass the right information down the chain.
- Consult with all the staff, identifying all the problems as they occur. Everybody underestimates the resources needed to put successful changes into place. You always need more people and more money than you thought you did at the beginning. Write down what resources you need, remembering to allow some extras for contingencies.
- Fix interval markers of progress to show you how far you have travelled on that journey towards your target. Feed the information back to the other people involved so that they can see how well everyone has done so far and look back on progress made. If you only get to look at the 'distant peak of the mountain' it never seems to get any nearer. You may find it helpful to fix up a few phone contacts or short meetings with your appraiser, or with a mentor or tutor, to measure your progress and get help with any blocks that you experience.
- Identify the threats. Make sure that other people do not feel threatened by what you propose. They need to feel they have a place and a role in the organisation or workplace. People should feel that what they do personally matters. Inevitably for some people, either yourself or the others involved in the modification to your working practice, the change will mean that what they are doing now will alter out of all recognition by the time the target is reached.

- Consider the chaos theory. We are working in organisations which are complex. A frequently quoted example of the chaos theory is that a butterfly flaps its wings on the other side of the world and sends all sorts of changes going through the atmosphere so that we have a thunderstorm here. Whatever we do has a knock-on effect. As soon as we start making one change, we need to anticipate the changes that are going to occur somewhere else, as far as possible. Beware of starting to make too many alterations at once.

Box 5.4:

Dr Frame decides that one of the practice nurses should take on a specialist role in secondary prevention, as part of his coronary heart disease prevention scheme. However, that will mean that she will have less time to share the care of the practice diabetic clinic, so he will need to plan who else is going to do that. At the same time another GP has plans to train the same practice nurse to set up a triage programme for emergency appointments. They discuss all the proposals with her and with the rest of the practice team. She is happy to take on some extra training for heart disease as it will fit in with her present skills and duties, but the practice team decide that they will have to bid for more funds to employ another nurse experienced in, or willing to train for, undertaking patient triage. The new post-holder will be able to take over some of the minor illness management from the other practice nurse. She can then spend more time running the diabetic clinic.

- Change can be hijacked by vested interests. Particular changes that are proposed are taken up for political reasons and changed again so that they are unrecognisable from the original version.
- The wrong target is chosen. You may be aiming for the wrong 'mountain' all along and, unfortunately, this often happens. You start a change and it is overtaken by other changes outside your control that make your original target incorrect or irrelevant.

Box 5.5:

Dr Aged is a general physician who decides that he needs to learn more about the management of elderly patients as he feels that he is not competent at caring for patients in older age groups. He starts his course of study, but a new hospital consultant is appointed who takes over the care of elderly patients, and puts into operation a programme of nurse specialist training to manage patients transferred to nursing homes.

- There may be a lack of commitment or failure to nominate deputies for action. We have all been to meetings where the key person with the critical piece of information for that meeting is not there and so the process stalls. You may have attended a meeting where hardly anyone turned up, so another had to be arranged before any progress could be made. There are one or two people without whom you cannot move forward; perhaps one of them is on sick leave and another on holiday, and the whole process grinds to a halt because those two are not there and have not handed on their responsibilities to deputies.

- Your changes may be sabotaged by external factors. You may find that you start on your action plan and all is going well for you personally – but then you receive a directive from your primary care organisation or hospital trust about a national priority that takes precedence.

- The resources and time that you were to obtain for implementing your PDP disappear, eaten up by a new priority from the trust. You need to make a fresh case to retain all or part of your plan and this delays its progress.

Personal reasons for resistance to change

You may be able to identify with some of the roles, described below, that people adopt when faced with change. If you can identify how you react, you can take this into consideration when drawing up your action plan. You might also find it helpful when discussing with others the modifications you want to make. Most of us have little bits of all of these reactions within us, but some fall mainly into one category and may have difficulties with moving forward because of their behaviour patterns.

- **Rebels** refuse to do things because someone in authority has suggested it. You probably know people who behave like two-year-olds when someone says, 'You need to do this,' and they think, 'Why should I?'. They may not link their reaction to the interaction that they used to have with authority figures in the past – perhaps a parent, a bossy teacher or a previous supervisor.

- **Oppressors** are very familiar too. They are often people with a little bit of authority who know 'how things should be done'. They may be at the stage of their own learning where they have not integrated the rules of how it should be done into a more flexible procedure of knowing what works from experience and expertise. They often expect specific actions to be taken without recognising what is important. There is a feeling of security in always following the same procedures and it can cover up the weakness that bullies often feel. It can also be laziness – an unwillingness to think about what they are doing or why it is done that way.

- **Victims** are helpless in the face of events. There are some people who whenever there is something to be done, or that needs to be altered, say,

'Oh, I suppose I'll have to do it'. They do it unwillingly and are not enthusiastic in taking it forward. They see it as something that is imposed upon them. They do not initiate the change or reflect on how it might be done better. They do not perceive themselves as being in charge of their own lives, or able to go out and get what they want. They usually have low self-esteem and cannot envisage anyone ever asking for, or taking notice of, their opinions.

- **Rescuers** always take the side of the victim and say, 'Oh, you don't really have to do that. There is some way we can get round it.' Rescuers may encourage people to ignore the necessity for change, to prevaricate and postpone actions that need to be taken. They often lack insight into the problem or knowledge about the dissatisfaction that led to the change being proposed. Although they may appear to be helping or supporting the person who has to make the changes, they can be subversive and undermine the forward momentum.

- **Overcautious** – another personal barrier to implementing your action plan can be due to a lack of frankness when providing your evidence and planning your objectives. This may have arisen through fear that being honest about your capabilities or your performance will lead to punitive action by the trust. If you have claimed that you already have a capacity to do something either personally or in supplying a service, then you cannot ask for help in achieving it as an objective in your development plan. If you believe that the trust will blame you personally for failures in the care of your patients when the problems really lie with a lack of resources or a gap in your knowledge or skills, you will not own up to that deficiency. It is important that appraisal fosters a supportive 'no-blame' culture, where sub-optimal performance can be reported as a problem to be rectified without a penalty being incurred. Appraisers, the lead clinician, clinical governance leads and chief executives all need to see underperformance as a multifaceted problem requiring assessment and then implementation of the solution, and not as an opportunity to penalise or vilify one part of the problem.

How to get help if you need it

Health professionals face many pressures. Many of these are common to most professional posts:

- meeting external standards (examinations, audit)
- competition (for resources, for staff, rivalries between specialties or individuals)
- information overload (keeping up to date, circulars, etc.)

- time management (there is always more work than time to do it in)
- financial (e.g. borrowing or bidding for money to finance improvements)
- relationship problems (at work and at home)
- career decisions (e.g. deciding whether to take on a committee, change direction or reduce commitments).

There are particular stressors which are more likely to occur in people working in a healthcare setting:

- coping with death and dying
- facing uncertainty because of the unpredictable nature of human beings
- making mistakes that could be fatal or serious
- lack of time and emotional resources for recreation, family and relationships.

Your problems are likely to fall into one of the following categories: academic, careers, professional, personal or administrative.

1 Academic support might include helping you to identify your learning needs and how you might meet them. You might ask for feedback and advice after examinations or audit activities, advice on study skills, or guidance on acquiring skills or knowledge. You might meet some of your needs by joining a group of your peers, asking for occasional advice from a tutor, or choosing to work with a mentor, clinical supervisor, coach or buddy. You might use a more formal framework organised by a specialist society or one of the specialist learning programmes supported by universities and other royal colleges. GPs may wish to use the Accredited Professional Development programme available from the Royal College of General Practitioners (*see* Appendix 1 for more information).

2 Careers support may include advice about alternatives to the present role, changes in direction or taking on or dropping commitments. You might seek advice or a sounding board from friends or colleagues, or from the supporting network you have for your academic work. Postgraduate deans and their educational teams are valuable sources of advice and support. Royal colleges are becoming increasingly active in supporting their members; the Royal College of Physicians has published an excellent vision of how it is going to provide even more career advice and support in the future.[3] Taking a sabbatical (or even just a holiday), or a short-term secondment post, may enable you to make a more informed decision.

3 You may benefit from professional counselling if your appraisal has identified deficiencies in your attitudes or behaviour. It may be that you need to learn to treat patients and colleagues with politeness and consideration. The appraiser, the senior clinician or clinical governance lead may recommend that you have help to develop knowledge of your limitations and increase your capacity for self-awareness.

4   Personal problems may include financial difficulties or relationship problems. You might ask, or be referred, for more specific counselling because of problems with your health, drug use or other difficulties.
5   Administrative problems mainly concern the organisation, the trust or the educational process. The appraiser may have sufficient information for you at the time, or you may need to contact your tutor, clinical lead or an administrative officer in the primary care organisation or hospital trust.

Assessing the quality of an appraisal

Appraisal originally came into the medical arena as an educational exercise to support and develop doctors in training. It is now more than that, but many issues about the quality of appraisal remain the same and the SCOPME (Standing Committee on Postgraduate Medical and Dental Education) criteria can be usefully applied to the appraisal process and experience of doctors in the UK. It is worth reflecting on your previous experiences of appraisal using the SCOPME checklists, substituting 'doctor' for 'trainee'. If your experience of appraisal has been negative then you may be able to identify why and how that could be rectified in the future.

Box 5.6:   SCOPME appraisal checklists[4]

Questions that judge discussion quality

- Are the appraisal discussions conducted in an atmosphere of trust?
- Are they held sufficiently often to meet trainees' needs and according to an agreed plan?
- Are they informed by a variety of assessments and other inputs?
- Are they conducted without interruption?
- Are they undertaken by an appraiser who works with the trainee, has been trained in appraisal, and is monitored in this role?
- Is there opportunity for self-appraisal by the trainee?
- Is there sufficient opportunity to review educational and personal matters, together with career ambitions?
- Are the interviews confidential to the appraiser and the trainee?
- Do they result in an agreed learning action plan and further learning opportunities as necessary?
- Is the learning reviewed regularly?

continued overleaf

Questions that judge scheme quality

- Is your appraisal system designed to identify educational and development needs of the trainee?
- Is it part of, and not a substitute for, day-to-day supervision, support and feedback about performance?
- Were trainees and trainers involved in devising, launching, implementing and reviewing your system?
- Is it recognised as separate from assessments conducted for regulatory purposes?
- Are the aims fully understood by all concerned?
- Is the system properly resourced?
- Do you have a mechanism for monitoring participation in appraisal?
- Do you have a mechanism for encouraging and collecting feedback about how well the system is working?
- Do you have a mechanism for reviewing your system and relaunching it as necessary?

Finally: make the time

In summary, what you are trying to set up when you go back into your workplace is a 'learning organisation', building innovation and flexibility into things that you do every day.[1,2] Protect the time – perhaps half a day every month – to step back from what you are doing to evaluate what's going on. Extract the learning points from what you do every day, day to day, to make plans for improvement for the future. Encourage suggestions from everybody in the workplace and facilitate individual development. This is a 'bottom-up' procedure – that is, not just accepting or resenting what other people with greater power or a higher position than you dictate, but actually thinking through for yourself what needs to be done.

References

1 Wakley G, Chambers R and Field S (2000) *Continuing Professional Development in Primary Care: making it happen.* Radcliffe Medical Press, Oxford.

2 Fisher A, Garcarz W, Chambers R and Nasir J (2002) *A Learning Organisation Strategy Template.* Staffordshire University, Stoke-on-Trent.

3 www.rcp.org.uk (accessed June 2002).

4 Oxley J (1997) Appraising doctors and dentists in training. *BMJ.* **315**: 2.

PART 2

Demonstrating the standards of your practice

Fashion your personal development plan and appraisal portfolio around *Good Medical Practice*

The work that you do for appraisal overlaps that required for revalidation, so the evidence recorded for appraisal will be available for revalidation as well. The General Medical Council sets out standards that must be met as part of the duties and responsibilities of doctors. In the booklet *Good Medical Practice* the General Medical Council introduces the contents by stating that:

'Patients must be able to trust doctors with their lives and well-being. To justify that trust, we as a profession have a duty to maintain a good standard of practice and to show respect for human life.'

The document points out that serious or persistent failure to meet the standards may put your registration at risk – not that most people would regard the standards as something to be achieved just because your job is on the line!

How will you demonstrate satisfactory standards?

The stages of the learning cycle for appraisal are given in Figure A. This learning cycle is common to all the aspects of appraisal and will be followed in each chapter.

Stage 1: setting standards and outcomes

Professional competence is the first area of concern in *Good Medical Practice*. You should be able to demonstrate that you can maintain a satisfactory standard

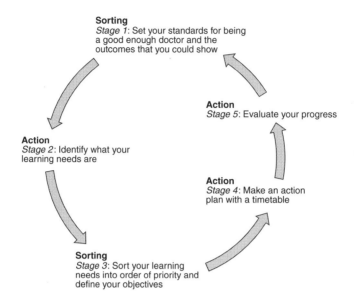

Sorting
Stage 1: Set your standards for being a good enough doctor and the outcomes that you could show

Action
Stage 5: Evaluate your progress

Action
Stage 2: Identify what your learning needs are

Action
Stage 4: Make an action plan with a timetable

Sorting
Stage 3: Sort your learning needs into order of priority and define your objectives

Figure A: The stages of the learning cycle for appraisal.

of clinical care most of the time. Some of the time you will be brilliant, of course! Celebrate those moments. On other occasions you or others will be critical of your performance and feel that you could have done much better. Reflect on those episodes to learn from them. The level at which you should be performing depends on your particular field of expertise. General practitioners are good at seeing the wider picture, specialists at being expert in a narrow area, so the level of competence in each area will vary. You would not, for example, expect orthopaedic specialists to be competent at managing cardiac failure (although some of them may be), but you would expect general practitioners to be able to manage all but the most complicated situations involving cardiac failure. You would expect both the orthopaedic specialist and the general practitioner to recognise the limits of their competence and refer to someone with more expertise when necessary.

Other standards include using resources effectively and the record-keeping that is an essential tool in clinical care. As a professional you need to be accessible and available so that you can provide your services and make suitable arrangements for handing over care to others. You must provide care in emergency situations.

By demonstrating your standards of practice around the seven main sections of *Good Medical Practice* you will organise your learning in the same format as that required for your appraisal paperwork. These seven sections and 'management' and 'research' are considered in depth in Chapters 6 to 14 inclusive.

Stage 2: identify your learning needs

Use methods to identify your learning that span several sections of the appraisal

You may decide to use a few selected methods to identify your learning needs in respect of 'good medical practice' that address the criteria in Box 6.1 that are also targeted at other topics or areas – included in the other sections of the GMC's booklet *Good Medical Practice*, mirrored within the appraisal forms. For this type of combined assessment, you might use:

- a self-assessment using a rating scale to assess your skills and attitudes, or peer review (*see* Chapter 6)
- a SWOT (strengths, weaknesses, opportunities and threats) analysis (*see* Chapter 7)
- other activities where you are keeping up to date (*see* Chapter 8)
- patient feedback or patient satisfaction surveys; significant event audit, constructive feedback with peer observation, 360° feedback, role description, or identifying team difficulties (*see* Chapter 9) to recognise where a lack of competence, accessibility or use of resources has affected the process or outcome for a patient
- areas where you are challenged during teaching and training to justify why you do what you do (*see* Chapter 10)
- evaluation of consent issues (*see* Chapter 11) to look at how you deal with issues of consent for examination, investigation or treatment and if patients' autonomy and right to decline is respected
- audit of protocols and guidelines (*see* Chapter 12) for checking how well procedures are followed; reviews of how resources, access and availability are managed
- review of patient records (*see* Chapter 13).

Stage 3: set your priorities and define your learning objectives

Group and summarise your learning needs from the exercises you have carried out. Grade them according to the priorities you set. You may put one at a higher priority because it fits in with learning needs established from another section, or put another lower because it does not fit in with other activities that you will put into your learning plan for the next 12 months. If you have identified a learning need by several different methods of assessment then it will have a higher priority than something identified only once.

Think about the following questions.

- Is your aim clear?
- Are you able to define your objectives?
- Can you justify spending time and effort on that topic? Is it serious enough or occurring sufficiently often to warrant the time spent?
- Are the time and resources for that topic available?
- Will learning about that topic make a difference to the care you can provide for patients?
- How does this topic fit in with other topics you have identified to learn more about?

Record what the learning needs assessments have contributed to establishing your needs, and which ones you have decided to concentrate on for now. Keep in mind that the health service exists to provide for the needs of patients.

Look back at Stage 1 of your standards taken from *Good Medical Practice*. Match your learning needs with one or more of these standards or others you have set yourself.

Stage 4: make an action plan with a timetable

Decide on what method of learning is most appropriate for your task. You may have already identified your preferred learning style – but *see* Chapter 10 for more information.

Describe how you will carry out your learning tasks and what you will do by a specified time. State how your learning will be applied and how and when it will be evaluated. Build in some staging posts so that you do not suddenly get to the end of 12 months and discover that you have only completed half of your plan.

Stage 5: evaluate your progress and disseminate the results

You might choose to evaluate and determine the outcome of your efforts by repeating the learning needs assessment that you started with. You might record your increased confidence in dealing with situations that you previously avoided or performed inadequately.

You could incorporate your assessment of what has been gained into a study of another area that overlaps.

6

Good medical practice

Stage 1: setting standards and outcomes

Look at the following criteria for good medical practice listed in Box 6.1. They are derived from *Good Medical Practice*.[1] You may want to add some others as well or expand the details given in Box 6.1. These describe the standards you will be showing that you meet in this section of the appraisal paperwork.

Box 6.1: Criteria for providing a good standard of practice and care

You should:

1 make an adequate assessment of the patient's condition, based on the history and, if indicated, an appropriate examination
2 provide or arrange investigations or treatment where necessary
3 take suitable and prompt action when required
4 be competent when making a diagnosis, and giving or arranging treatment
5 recognise and work within the limits of your competence
6 refer to another practitioner when indicated
7 consult with colleagues and keep them informed when sharing the care of patients
8 keep clear, legible and contemporaneous records that include the clinical findings, decisions made, information given to patients and any treatments given or prescribed
9 provide necessary care to alleviate pain and distress whether or not curative treatment is possible
10 give treatment only where you have adequate knowledge of the patient's health and medical needs
11 recommend or give investigations or treatment only when in the best interests of the patient, but not withhold them inappropriately
12 report adverse drug reactions and co-operate with organisations requiring information to monitor the public health, keeping in mind the confidentiality of patient information
13 make efficient use of resources, but record, report and endeavour to rectify deficiencies in resources

continued overleaf

---

14 not allow your beliefs to affect the advice or treatment you provide, or if your beliefs are likely to affect your patient management, tell patients of their right to see another doctor

15 give priority to the care of patients on the basis of clinical need

16 offer anyone at risk in an emergency the assistance you could reasonably be expected to provide

17 not refuse to treat a patient because of personal risk, but take reasonable steps to protect yourself before providing care.

Stage 2: identify your learning needs

Choose your methods of identifying your learning needs to determine how standards of your own practice compare with the criteria given in *Good Medical Practice*.

You could use:

- self-assessment using a rating scale to assess your skills and attitudes
- peer review
- reflective practice identifying your learning needs or patients' needs by recording from each consultation what you left out from lack of awareness, or what you forgot or deliberately withheld, and whether that consultation met the patient's needs or not
- keeping a diary or a case report of a patient who requires continuity of care.

These four methods are described in more detail below.

(i) Self-assessment using a rating scale

Self-assessment has been criticised as being inaccurate, but it can be a useful tool in establishing areas where you do not feel confident. A paper from Auckland examined the ability of doctors to assess their own levels of knowledge over a variety of subjects.[2] The accuracy was tested against a 'true–false' written test. The authors concluded that the correlation was too poor for self-assessment to be used for professional development programmes. However, it is difficult to know how relevant some of the test questions were. Recall of information, or access to recently published work, is likely to be low in an area where interest has not been promoted by the recent presentation of a patient with that particular problem. Doctors are adult learners used to selecting what and when they learn. Given the opportunity, adults will choose topics relevant to their work at a level appropriate to their current knowledge.[3]

You might draw up a list of skills that are relevant to your job, or use one that has already been developed for use in training situations.[4] Many trainees are assessed in this way when first starting a job so that they and their trainers can draw up an initial learning programme.

Box 6.2:

Dr Peep filled in a rating scale about how confident he was in using all the equipment in his consulting room. He realised that he had never felt at ease using an ophthalmoscope and was not really sure what he should be looking for when examining the retina – he just hoped he would recognise something abnormal when he saw it. All the other equipment in the room was in frequent use and he felt confident that he used everything else correctly and with skill. He recorded his need to add retinoscopy to his learning plan.

It is probably easier to assess yourself regarding how you use your skills in practical ways than establishing your level of confidence in your patient management skills, clinical judgement, time management or professional values, etc. However, spending some time reflecting on all the parameters of your job might enable you to see some gaps, or to appreciate that there are areas you had not previously considered as relevant. You may want to follow up your self-assessment with other checks by peer review or more objective measures.

If you work in general practice, you can compare how often you manage specific problems (from very rarely to very frequently) with data from practices that contribute to the Office of Population Censuses and Surveys' dataset.[5] If your ratings are very different, consider if it is because you are not competent in those fields or whether your practice is unusual.

You might also look to see how well you rate your knowledge and ability to manage each condition. You might draw up a list where you rate your need to increase your ability to deal with common conditions. Consider also, if a condition is rare, is it of such importance that it is a high priority that you should manage it well? Your assessment of your management of a condition might include:

- assessment and diagnosis
- providing or arranging investigations
- providing or arranging treatment
- emergency treatment
- identifying where the limits of your competence lie and when you should refer
- what records you keep
- prevention of that condition.

(ii) Peer review

The JoHari Window is a useful concept to understand the function of feedback from others in the identification of both strengths and learning needs. Box 6.3 illustrates the idea that there are areas unknown to yourself but known to others.

Box 6.3: JoHari Window	
I **Public area** Known to others Known to self	II **Blind area** Known to others Not known to self
III **Avoided or hidden area** Not known to others Known to self	IV **Area of unknown activity** Not known to others Not known to self

Note: The JoHari Window is named after Jo Luft and Harry Ingham, not Johari!

During appraisal, the public area (I) will increase as you reveal or demonstrate parts of area III. Peer review, appraisal and other activities to determine your learning needs will decrease the size of areas II and IV.

Box 6.4: JoHari Window after peer review or appraisal	
I **Public area** Known to others Known to self	II **Blind area** Known to others Not known to self
III **Avoided or hidden area** Not known to others Known to self	IV **Area of unknown activity** Not known to others Not known to self

Challenge from other people or external factors reduces quadrant IV and increases the size of quadrants I and II. Internal monitoring also helps to reduce the size of quadrants II and IV, so that qualities, skills or abilities in these areas can become uncovered and moved to quadrants I or III.

There is universal curiosity about quadrants III and IV but this is held in check by custom, social training and fear of what might be revealed. We all need to be sensitive to the covert aspects in quadrants II, III and IV and respect the desire of individuals to keep them hidden.

A number of surgical specialties, with cardiothoracic surgery leading the way, have outcome measures which are held on national registers and can be used to compare a surgeon's performance against others, adjusted for case mix. This information is hard evidence and is definitely in the public area (I) of the JoHari Window. If a surgeon is asked the question, 'How do you know you are competent?' the surgeon can reply, 'I am on the 53rd centile of surgeons in my specialty for mortality for this particular operation.' This is fine if the surgeon is near average, but the lower centiles have to be interpreted with caution as generally small numbers of cases are being performed in statistical terms, and a run of bad luck can be interpreted by the statistically naive as evidence of underperformance.

You might work with someone as a pair so that each of you can benefit from the peer review – but be careful that you don't end up as a cosy couple colluding in ignoring each other's defects! On the other hand, constant criticism will be demoralising and reduce your motivation, so remember to resist the temptation to launch straight into what has been omitted or not done well. Always start by feeding back and reinforcing what has been done well or adequately. Make your feedback fit the mnemonic **SMART**.

- **S**pecific.
- **M**easurable.
- **A**ttainable.
- **R**elevant.
- **T**ime-signalled.

Box 6.5:

Dr Level and Dr Exact agreed to assess each other's skill base before taking on the teaching of undergraduates. Dr Level took several blood pressure readings under observation. His feedback included that he explained the procedure and the significance of the results well – but that he often did not support the arm at the level of the heart and did not use a large enough cuff.[6] Dr Exact did his joint injection with Dr Level assisting.[7] He was good at explaining the procedure and established a good doctor–patient relationship. He was skilful and quick but careless about cross-infection. They were surprised how careless each had become about such basic skills. They had forgotten the principles underlying the skills and got into the habit of performing them rapidly and without due regard to accuracy or safety.

(iii) Reflective practice

A well-established way of reflecting on your daily practice and discovering your learning needs is *Learning with PUNs and DENs*.[8] The essential part of consulting with a patient is discovering what his or her needs are by making a diagnosis. If you are unable to meet that patient's need (for information, treatment, understanding, etc.) then a **P**atient's **U**nmet **N**eed (PUN) is recorded. This leads to a **D**octor's **E**ducational **N**eed (DEN). If that educational need is met the next time the doctor meets that particular patient's need, it can be fulfilled. It is easy to keep a running diary after each consultation to record these. Then you need to reflect whether to try to meet that need entirely from your own resources (e.g. by learning a new skill or acquiring some new knowledge) or if it would be better dealt with by delegation or referral.

(iv) Keeping a diary or a case report

Patients often encounter poor care when their illness is not one short episode or requires multidisciplinary support. You could monitor your standards of care in chronic illness, disabilities and terminal care by recording chrono-logically what happens to the patient. Sharing this account at a clinical meeting would help you to be aware of any gaps in the management that you had not previously identified. This might also assist in discovering needs for working with colleagues or managing resources better.

Stage 3: set your priorities and define your learning objectives

You might have found out that the way investigations are carried out in your department or practice is haphazard and poorly organised. Your objective might be to provide a paper or computer folder with a summary entry for each investigation: where it is performed, how it can be arranged and how the results are communicated to the patient. You may need to learn more about using the computer to be able to reach this objective.

A peer review may have shown that your resuscitation skills are rusty and out of date. Your objective may be to attend a relevant course and pass the assessment at the end of it to show that you are competent.

A record of your reflective learning may show that you have little know-ledge of the voluntary societies that can give support to patients. Your object-ive would be to ask one of the secretaries to collect data about local contacts for voluntary societies and make details available as a resource on the computer for all of the team.

A case study may reveal that poor symptom control in a patient with terminal illness was partly due to your lack of knowledge and partly due to lack of communication with the district nurses and the hospice nurse. Your objective will be to show up-to-date knowledge of symptom control and clearer lines of communication between the members of the team who care for terminally ill patients.

Stage 4: make an action plan with a timetable

A simple Gantt chart like that in Figure 6.1 helps you to track what you are going to do and when. For example, you may want to improve your management of sexually transmitted infections (STIs).[9]

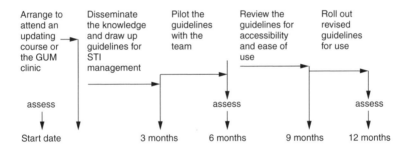

Figure 6.1:   A Gantt chart for your action plan – good medical practice.

Stage 5: evaluate your progress and disseminate the results

You might choose to evaluate and determine the outcome of your efforts by repeating the learning needs assessment(s) with which you started. You might record your increased confidence in dealing with situations that you previously avoided or performed inadequately. You might value the peer review from colleagues about your improved skills or attitudes. A new case study about a patient might show better care and fewer problems.

You could incorporate your assessment of what has been gained into a study of another area that overlaps – perhaps as detailed in Chapter 7 for maintaining good practice or one of the subsequent chapters.

EXAMPLE DIARY SHEETS FOR THIS SECTION

Diary sheet for section on good medical practice EXAMPLE 1	
Stage 1: criteria and outcomes selected	To show that this doctor: 1 makes an adequate assessment of the patient's condition based on the history and appropriate examination 2 provides or arranges investigations where necessary.
Stage 2: methods of assessment	1 Comparison of diagnosis of patient with findings at operation. 2 Peer review of relevance of, and indications for, investigations.
Stage 3: which objectives have been selected for action this year and why	Practitioner's reviews showed diagnoses did differ from findings at operation sometimes, and investigations were ordered unnecessarily. The objectives are to: • seek out and trial computer-aided diagnostic pathways to improve accuracy of diagnosis to avoid unnecessary or incorrect operative procedures • draw up clearer guidelines on the use of 'routine' investigations performed by junior staff to increase the relevance of those performed.
Stage 4: the action plan	Baseline assessment as above. By 3 months: obtain information on computer-aided packages and draw up draft guidelines on investigation relevance. By 6 months: finish pilot studies on both. At 9 months: apply revised packages and guidelines. At 12 months: reapply assessment and analyse results.
Stage 5: evaluation of progress	1 Discussion of use of draft guidelines at 3 months and implementation of pilot use of guidelines on investigations. 2 Practise using computer-aided diagnostic aid for one condition and assess its usefulness personally and for the team. 3 Guidelines incorporated into reference resource for junior staff.

Diary sheet for section on good medical practice
EXAMPLE 2

Stage 1: criteria and outcomes selected	To show that this doctor: 1 consults with colleagues and keeps them informed 2 keeps adequate and clear records.
Stage 2: methods of assessment	1 Case studies of three diabetic patients who have other chronic medical conditions and whose care is shared. 2 Case record review of the medication of patients with diabetes whose care is shared with other health professionals.
Stage 3: which objectives have been selected for action this year and why	Medication on the shared record card is not always clear or accurate at present. Objective is to: • ensure that medication is updated • agree roles and responsibilities within team.[10]
Stage 4: the action plan	Baseline assessment as above. By 3 months: meet with all (or representatives from) the groups of professionals involved in the shared care. By 6 months: trial of a computer print-out of medication issued each time the patient is seen in the general practice and inserted into a plastic sleeve in the shared care record. Dated and signed amendments made by hand by health professionals when the patient is seen elsewhere. Meeting with patients arranged to involve them in the plan. At 9 months: review of progress, meeting with staff involved, meeting with patients. Patients very enthusiastic and are reminding the staff to complete the record. At 12 months: reapply assessment and analyse. Feedback to staff and patients.
Stage 5: evaluation of progress	1 Review of progress by verbal feedback from staff and patients at the meetings. 2 Review of shared records at 9 and 12 months.

References

1   General Medical Council (2001) *Good Medical Practice*. General Medical Council, London.

2   Tracey JM, Arroll B, Richmond DE *et al.* (1997) The validity of general practitioners' self-assessment of knowledge: cross sectional study. *BMJ.* **315**: 1426–8.

3   Tough AM (1979) *The Adult's Learning Projects; a fresh approach to theory and practice in adult learning.* Research in education, series 1. Ontario Institute for Studies in Education, Toronto.

4   Chambers R (ed.) (2002) *A Guide to Accredited Professional Development: pathway to revalidation.* Royal College of General Practitioners, London.

5   Office of Population Censuses and Surveys (1995) *Morbidity Statistics from General Practice: fourth national study 1991–2 series MB5 no. 3.* HMSO, London.

6   Chambers R, Wakley G and Iqbal Z (2001) *Cardiovascular Disease Matters in Primary Care.* Radcliffe Medical Press, Oxford.

7   Wakley G, Chambers R and Dieppe P (2001) *Musculoskeletal Matters in Primary Care.* Radcliffe Medical Press, Oxford.

8   Eve R (1994) *Learning with PUNs and DENs.* R Eve, Taunton.

9   Wakley G and Chambers R (2001) *Sexual Health Matters in Primary Care.* Radcliffe Medical Press, Oxford.

10 Chambers R, Stead J and Wakley G (2001) *Diabetes Matters in Primary Care.* Radcliffe Medical Press, Oxford.

7

Maintaining good medical practice

Introduction

This is the section in which doctors with special interests may focus on particular topics relating to their expertise. For instance, GPs with special interests (GPwSIs) or consultants developing new skills can demonstrate attaining and maintaining their expert status here.

How will you demonstrate satisfactory standards?

Remind yourself of the stages of the learning cycle for appraisal (*see* Figure A).

Stage 1: setting standards and outcomes

Look at the following criteria for maintaining medical practice listed in Box 7.1. They are derived from *Good Medical Practice*.[1] You may want to add some others as well or expand the details given in Box 7.1. These describe the

---

Box 7.1: Criteria for maintaining good medical practice

You should:

1 keep your knowledge and skills up to date throughout your working life, through continuing educational activities which maintain and develop your competence and performance
2 keep up to date with the laws and statutory codes of practice which affect your work

continued overleaf

3 work with colleagues to monitor and maintain the quality of care you provide
4 be continually aware of patient safety
5 take part in regular and systematic medical and clinical audits and make improvements accordingly
6 respond constructively to the outcomes of reviews, assessments or appraisals of your performance
7 take part in confidential enquiries, and adverse event recognition and reporting, to help reduce risk to patients.

standards you will be showing that you meet in this section of the appraisal paperwork.

Stage 2: identify your learning needs

Choose your methods of identifying your learning needs to determine how standards of your own practice compare with the criteria given in *Good Medical Practice*.

You could:

- undertake an audit of protocols and guidelines
- carry out an analysis of your strengths, weaknesses, opportunities and threats (SWOT)
- review whether you are employing appropriate methods of learning for the nature of the topics or skills you need to learn about.

These three methods are described in more detail below.

(i) Audit of protocols and guidelines

Audit is about setting standards for your performance, finding out how you are doing, searching to find out best practice, making the changes and then re-auditing the care given to patients in the future with the same problem.[2]

Audit can be any of the following.

- Case-note analysis. This provides insight into current practice described in protocols or guidelines. It can be a retrospective review of a random selection of notes, or a prospective survey of consecutive patients with the same condition.
- Criteria-based audit. This compares clinical practice with specific standards, guidelines or protocols. A re-audit of changes should demonstrate improvements in the quality of patient care. You could measure how well

your care of patients is managed by comparing the proportion of patients meeting your criteria for good care over intervals of time. Consult with all those involved – the patients and carers, nurses, doctors, reception staff, therapists, pharmacists etc. – to improve what you do, put it into action and then re-audit.

• External audit. Audit facilitators, prescribing advisers, training and development managers etc. can all supply information about indicators of performance which may be useful in carrying out an audit. However, the team has to be involved and use the information in an audit capacity. Visits from external bodies, such as those linked to accreditation by the royal colleges or Commission for Health Improvement, expose trusts and individual practitioners to external audit.

Box 7.2:
Dr Red organised an audit of the timeliness of thrombolytic drugs given to people admitted to an accident and emergency department with chest pain. Each time a thrombolytic drug was administered, the event was recorded. One month on, the team reviewed the results and compared them with the standard described in the protocol for their A&E unit. They found that they were doing well and met their standard; a re-audit was entered in the diary for a year's time.

(ii) An analysis of your strengths, weaknesses, opportunities and threats (SWOT)[3]

You can undertake a SWOT analysis of your own performance or that of your team in your department, practice or trust. Brainstorm the strengths, weaknesses, opportunities and threats of the situation on your own, or with a workmate or mentor, or with a group of colleagues.

Strengths and weaknesses of individual practitioners might include: knowledge, experience, expertise, decision-making, communication skills, interprofessional relationships, political skills, timekeeping, organisational skills, teaching skills and research skills. Strengths and weaknesses of the department, practice or trust might relate to most of these aspects too, as well as resources – staff, skills, structural parts.

Opportunities might relate to unexploited potential strengths, expected changes, options for career development pathways, and hobbies or interests that might usefully be expanded.

Threats will include factors and circumstances that prevent you from achieving your aims for personal, professional and practice development.

Prioritise important factors. Draw up a list of goals and a timed action plan to make the most of strengths and opportunities and combat weaknesses and threats.

(iii) Review of whether you are employing appropriate methods of learning

People choose to learn in ways that they are used to, or that are most convenient, rather than in the most appropriate way for the topic they need to learn about. They usually opt for the mode of learning or training with which they are most familiar (usually a lecture or validated professional course) or which is most suited to their working conditions. Review whether you have matched your educational requirements for the last twelve months with the mode of delivery that was most appropriate for the topic you had planned to learn about – e.g. in last year's personal development plan or at your last appraisal. You might discuss this review with a peer as described in Chapter 6.

Stage 3: set your priorities and define your learning objectives

You might find that the audit of your clinical protocol showed that you were achieving the standards set – but even so you may choose to improve your performance further. Your objective might be to learn to delegate or to teach others to assume new roles and responsibilities within a particular clinical protocol; or it could involve you learning relevant skills or increasing the efficiency or effectiveness of your systems at work.

A SWOT analysis of an aspect of maintaining good medical practice – such as if a review, assessment or appraisal has revealed problems in your performance – might focus on your weaknesses in a new area such as patient and public involvement. Your objective might be to learn how to explain risks to patients or involve them in decision-making.

A review of your methods of learning might have revealed that you are stuck in a rut, only going to lectures – this may be an inappropriate way of learning. You set your objective to make more of distance learning and electronic sources – but first you have to learn to download and operate a CD-ROM or navigate around websites.

Stage 4: make an action plan with a timetable

A simple Gantt chart like that in Figure 7.1 helps you to track what you are going to do and when.

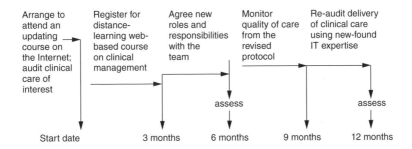

Figure 7.1:   A Gantt chart for your action plan – maintaining good medical practice.

Stage 5: evaluate your progress and disseminate the results

You might choose to evaluate and determine the outcome of your efforts by repeating the learning needs assessment(s) that you started with.

You could incorporate your assessment of what has been gained into a study of another area that overlaps – perhaps as detailed in Chapter 6 for good medical practice or one of the following chapters.

References

1   General Medical Council (2001) *Good Medical Practice*. General Medical Council, London.

2   National Institute for Clinical Excellence (2002) *Principles for Best Practice in Clinical Audit*. Radcliffe Medical Press, Oxford.

3   Wakley G and Chambers R (2000) *Continuing Professional Development: making it happen*. Radcliffe Medical Press, Oxford.

EXAMPLE DIARY SHEET FOR THIS SECTION

Diary sheet for section on maintaining good medical practice	
Stage 1: criteria and outcomes selected	To show that this doctor: 1 works with colleagues to monitor and maintain the quality of care they provide 2 maintains and develops their competence.
Stage 2: methods of assessment	1 Audits a particular aspect of clinical care, comparing standards with current protocol. 2 Undertakes a SWOT analysis of way in which care defined by clinical protocol is delivered.
Stage 3: which objectives have been selected for action this year and why	1 Audit shows that many patients are not complying with treatment plans. 2 SWOT analysis concludes that nurses could be substituted for doctors at many of the stages in the clinical protocol. 3 Review shows that doctor could make more use of e-learning sources. The objectives are to: • revise the clinical protocol so that patients are involved in decision-making about treatment options • substitute nurses for doctors wherever possible while maintaining patient safety • learn more about e-learning to be able to make use of its full potential.
Stage 4: the action plan	Baseline assessment as above and delegate collection of data about patient outcomes at various stages of clinical protocol. By 3 months: register for a web-based course. By 6 months: meet with clinical team to discuss and plan revisions to clinical protocol. Business plan still under discussion with management. At 9 months: monitor whether quality of care is improved; review whether nurses who have substituted for doctors have further training needs. At 12 months: re-audit delivery of clinical care according to revised protocol.
Stage 5: evaluation of progress	1 Review of progress by verbal interchange of information with staff at meetings. 2 Meetings with manager to receive progress reports from re-audit and patient feedback. 3 Assessment from e-learning course.

8

Relationships with patients

Introduction

When people present themselves as patients, they do so in the expectation (usually) that they can trust the health professionals to do their best for them. The concept of becoming a 'patient' has often meant that someone loses the status as a human being able to act independently. Better health and stability are often bought at an excessive price of loss of autonomy, particularly in a hospital setting. All health professionals need to strive towards continuing as members of the wider society. They have to reject the autocratic role often instilled by hierarchical hospital training and become responsible not only towards themselves and their superiors, but also to the patients and the people, the whole community. Patients must be free to reach for their own responsibilities, identify and analyse the situation, and face the reality of their own condition. The specialist information that health professionals have has to be balanced against the intimate knowledge of self that each person possesses.

Our own reactions and attitudes to people can prove to be a problem. The impact on us of severe disfigurement, incontinence, severe speech impairments or hearing loss may hamper our ability to fulfil some of the roles outlined below, and it is important that we are aware of our own problems and prejudices. We often make premature judgements about people that can affect the way we behave.

Remember to think about each patient as an individual who has a life outside the surgery or clinic where you are consulting. The appearance people present may give non-verbal clues about their attitude to life, but may be seriously misleading. Putting people into categories because of their culture, religion or accent can be just as unhelpful. It is sometimes difficult to balance professional and personal roles, particularly for those who work in small communities where their personal lives are common knowledge. In any situation, it is essential to guard against exploiting the power imbalance between patient and physician by exerting undue influence. The dependence, transference or gratitude that some patients may show needs to be balanced by a proper professional attitude.

Box 8.1:

Dr Kleen tried to control her annoyance. The young man sitting by the desk was wearing torn jeans and a faded T-shirt. If anything, the girl with him looked even less well-cared for in a limp skirt and voluminous sweater. He had just announced, 'She needs a letter for the housing.' The doctor said firmly, 'Tell me what the medical problem is; I can't just write a letter.' To her surprise, she heard a story about how the girl had been taken in off the streets by this young man, after her parents had thrown her out. He only knew her a little, and was not the father of the child she was carrying – the reason for her expulsion from her home by a dominating and unforgiving father. The doctor found herself sharing with this unkempt young man a sense of responsibility for the needs of this vulnerable girl.

You could consider the following concepts.

- *Partnership*: help for people who are ill or disabled comes through partnerships between patients and healthcare professionals.[1]
- *Empowerment*: our role is to help empower those with ailments to find the best ways of helping themselves, not impose solutions on them.
- *Judgement*: beware of judgement – the patient with the problem is the one who really understands his or her experience and problems.
- *Values*: people's values and priorities change with time; they may be quite different from your current values, but are no less valid.
- *Assumptions*: do not assume that you know how people feel or think, or that you know what they believe. Always check your understanding before proceeding. People interpret their belief systems, their culture and life experiences in many ways.
- *Autonomy*: autonomy should be a fundamental right of everyone. Illness or disability can mean a loss of some aspects of autonomy in society.
- *Listening*: this is the most important word for health professionals. Active, non-judgemental listening is the core art of medicine and crucial to gaining an understanding of people with illness or disabilities.
- *Shared decision-making*: people with chronic conditions need to be able to take their own decisions about their management, based on the expert information communicated to them by health professionals. Shared decision-making leads to concordance.
- *Concordance*: a negotiated agreement on treatment between the patient and the healthcare professional allows patients to take informed decisions on the degree of risk or suffering that they themselves wish to undertake or follow.[2] In contrast, 'compliance' with treatment or lifestyle changes implies that the patient follows instructions from health professionals to a greater or lesser degree – usually the latter.

Collecting evidence of good relationships with patients

In the hospital service there will be systems in place for collecting and responding to complaints as part of the governance arrangements. In addition, databases will be developed that list complaints within a directorate or a division and these databases can be interrogated to identify which complaints relate to an individual clinician. That data is likely to be brought to appraisal meetings in the future and needs to be balanced. We are relatively good at responding to adverse criticism, in that we take it seriously, even if we do not like it! We are generally poor at responding to praise. We dismiss it and get embarrassed. In order to balance the collation of criticism, some directorates have started collating letters of praise from patients. Clinicians would be well advised to collect individual letters from grateful patients and use them as evidence of good relationships. When patients come to clinic singing the praises of the care they received on the ward or from the practice team – yes, it does happen – a hint to them to drop a line to the chief executive or practice manager may be a good idea. A verbal statement by a patient can be turned into a durable piece of evidence to be used in appraisal.

How will you demonstrate satisfactory standards?

Remind yourself of the stages of the learning cycle for appraisal (*see* Figure A).

Stage 1: setting standards and outcomes

You might include some of the following criteria of a good relationship with patients, listed in Box 8.2, that are derived from *Good Medical Practice*.[3] You may want to add some others as well.

You do not have to provide detailed outcomes for *all* of the standards you have set in Stage 1. You may well find that some of them naturally appear as part of your continuing need to keep up to date (*see* Chapter 6) or in other sections.

Many of the learning outcomes for relationships with patients overlap with criteria for working with colleagues (Chapter 9), demonstrating probity (Chapter 11), management activity (Chapter 12) and other requirements.

Box 8.2: Criteria for a good relationship with patients

You should:

1 treat patients with courtesy and consideration
2 treat all patients equally and ensure that some groups are not favoured at the expense of others
3 be aware of how personal beliefs can affect the care offered to the patient, and take care not to impose beliefs and values on patients who may have alternative views
4 maintain the patient's dignity, especially during physical examination
5 obtain informed consent to physical examination, investigations and treatment
6 respect the autonomy of the patient to refuse examination, investigations or treatment
7 inform patients and carers about their condition in a way that they can understand
8 empower patients to take decisions about their management
9 keep information about patients confidential and explain the necessity of confidentiality to others
10 seek consent before sharing information; consult or discuss patients where confidential information cannot be overheard
11 avoid situations where personal and professional interests might be in conflict, or where one might influence the other overtly or covertly, especially if personal advantage might be achieved
12 apologise appropriately when things go wrong, and have an adequate complaint procedure in place
13 be able to justify why ending a professional relationship with a patient is fair and communicate those reasons to the patient.

Box 8.3:

Dr Wright struggled to find any good simple leaflets on fungal infections of the skin. He was learning about these conditions as part of his development plan to increase his knowledge and skills in dermatology. He found a good one by searching on the internet, but it was couched in very American-sounding English. He rewrote it, and then asked for feedback from his patients on a short questionnaire. After some minor alterations, he put it into the bank of patient leaflets available to all the health professionals in his workplace. He also gave a talk about fungal conditions at a meeting and found his leaflet very well received by other health professionals. He was able to record that he met the criteria 7 and 8 from the list in Box 8.2.

Stage 2: identify your learning needs

You may decide to incorporate your learning needs assessment for relationships with patients together with one of the other areas, so that you cover more than one in a single assessment. For this type of combined assessment, you might use:

- significant event audit (*see* Chapter 9) for identifying whether communication problems or consultation skills contributed to a problem
- audit of protocols and guidelines (*see* Chapter 12) for checking how well confidentiality procedures are followed
- structured peer observation (*see* Chapter 9) for feedback on your communication skills from other health workers such as doctors, nurses, receptionists and secretaries
- self-assessment (*see* Chapter 6) using a rating scale to assess your skills and attitudes in consultation
- evaluation of consent issues (*see* Chapter 11) to look at how you deal with issues of consent for examination, investigation or treatment and if patients' autonomy and right to decline is respected
- examination of patient records (*see* Chapter 13) to determine what information you have not managed to obtain that might be of significance in the management of those patients and to formulate reasons and remedies for why you have not done so
- patient complaint reviews (*see* Chapter 12) to identify the communication problems that have led to a complaint being made.

Learning needs assessment techniques that are particularly suitable for use in determining standards in relationships with patients are:

- patient feedback
- patient satisfaction surveys
- audio or videotape review of consultations
- seminar review of consultations and reflective feedback.

These four methods are described in more detail below.

(i) Patient feedback

Some general information can be gathered from national surveys of NHS services for patients and what patients say they want from health professionals. The publication *Health Which* from the Consumer Association often has articles that are of relevance to doctors and nurses consulting or giving information, and looks at the situation from the consumer's point of view. Although this publication tries to obtain a cross-sectional approach, keep in mind that it will inevitably be a little biased towards middle-class aspirations and may not be applicable to the patients in your area without modification. The Commission for Health Improvement collects patient experiences and comments and these will be fed back to you after an inspection. You can access collections of the experiences of patients with certain conditions from the link on the National Electronic Library of Medicine homepage (*see* Appendix 1).

Suggestion boxes can be the source of surprising comments. To increase the usefulness of these, you have to build in a method of informing patients about comments that have been made and what action has been taken. A box that seems a black hole into which pieces of paper drop, never to be seen again, is not a good incentive. The staff on reception desks can be a good influence, encouraging the use of the boxes as a source of positive suggestions, not just the moans.

Record individual comments and collect cards of appreciation – they can help to reinforce the good aspects of your consultation skills and relationships, and may demonstrate a trend or theme that you want to take up and develop.

You might identify how difficult it is to obtain meaningful information about patients' views and incorporate that into your learning plan.

If you have a patients' forum, or have set up a focus group, its feedback needs to be examined to establish how representative it is. It is easy for groups to be hijacked by vociferous enthusiasts.

(ii) Patient satisfaction surveys

One person, such as the practice or ward manager, clerical assistant or secretary, should take charge of the organisation of patient satisfaction surveys. In order to ensure that information from different places is comparable, and that changes can be monitored, it is essential that the survey is undertaken in a standardised manner and that all staff involved know what to do.

It is preferable to use a questionnaire that has been tried and tested previously. Designing your own questionnaire risks including flawed and ambiguous questions that may give misleading results. The results from a tested questionnaire are more likely to be valid and reliable, and it will save you a lot of time. The results can be compared with those previously obtained and can be used to show change. The results can also be compared with those obtained by other health professionals using the same questionnaire – so that you can compare your results with theirs. Some questionnaires already available are listed opposite and further details about how to apply and evaluate them are given in the following pages. You can use the results to discuss with colleagues in what ways you might need to alter your consultation style.

LIST OF SOME OF THE QUESTIONNAIRES AVAILABLE

1 The Doctors' Interpersonal Skills Questionnaire (DISQ) is designed to give GPs structured patient feedback on their interpersonal skills within consultations. It contains 12 items that include listening and explanation skills, warmth of greeting, respect for the patient and whether the patient has been able to express his or her concerns or fears. Patients can add their comments on how doctors can improve their services. It has been validated and used widely in several countries. You would need to arrange for 50 consecutive patients to be given the questionnaire to complete after a consultation with you. It takes just a few minutes to complete and post in a box at the reception desk. The practice sends the completed questionnaires back to Exeter University for analysis and results. The results are presented in a format giving structured patient feedback and comparisons with results from over 2000 GPs working in the UK.

2 The Patient Enablement Instrument (PEI) consists of a short questionnaire (as in Box 8.4). It can be used without permission, but you will need to obtain details about how it should be administered and scored in Howie et al.[4]

Box 8.4: Patient Enablement Instrument

As a result of this visit to the doctor today, do you feel you are:

1	able to cope with life?	Much more	More	Same or less
2	able to understand your illness?	Much more	More	Same or less
3	able to cope with your illness?	Much more	More	Same or less
4	able to keep yourself healthy?	Much more	More	Same or less
5	confident about your health?	Much more	More	Same or less
6	able to help yourself?	Much more	More	Same or less

---

3 The General Practice Assessment Survey (GPAS-2) is available by downloading it from the website (www.gpas.co.uk) together with a manual of how it can be used and scored. It is free to use but always acknowledge the source. It measures communication and interpersonal care including listening, explaining, time, caring and patience, as well as how well the doctor knows the patient, enablement and referral. It also includes scores for access and availability, receptionists, continuity of care and practice nursing care – these would be useful for your management and working with colleague requirements as well. It records socio-economic details so that the results can be compared across practices or trusts. It takes about five minutes to complete and can be given out in the surgery or sent by post. The National Primary Care Research and Development Centre (NPCRDC) at the University of Manchester provides a

service to analyse and report on GPAS-2 data for primary care organisations.

4   The Patient Satisfaction Questionnaire (PSQ) includes 20 items relating to patient satisfaction with doctors, as well as eight items on access, four each on appointments, facilities and nurses, plus a separate six-item scale to measure general satisfaction with the service provided by the practice. Details are given in Grogan *et al.*[5]

5   The Patient Experience Questionnaire (PEQ) was developed in Norwegian primary care. It has 14 items written as statements; patients complete the questionnaire by marking their degree of agreement with the statements on a five-point Likert scale from 'agree strongly' to 'disagree strongly'. It includes statements about the outcome of a specific visit, the communication and barriers to communication, and experiences with auxiliary staff. Details have been published in Steine *et al.*[6]

6   DIALOGUE, available from the Department of General Practice at the University of Leicester, consists of two questionnaires. The Surgery Satisfaction Questionnaire (SSQ) asks patients for their opinions on the service provided by the practice as a whole. The questions concern six components of care – general satisfaction, accessibility (getting to the surgery), availability of care (i.e. appointments, telephone answering), continuity, opinions on medical care, and premises. The Consultation Satisfaction Questionnaire (CSQ) asks patients for their opinions of the consultation. The questions concern four components of care – general satisfaction with the consultation, opinions on the professional aspects of the consultation, the depth of the relationship and the perceived duration of the consultation.

5   Other questionnaires have been developed in the USA. Have a look at the websites of the American Board of Internal Medicine or the Physician Review programme. However, many of these contain enquiries about financing or information that is hospital- or clinic-specific (*see* Appendix 1).

6   Patient satisfaction questionnaires have been developed by some of the royal colleges and are particularly relevant to specialties. Make sure that they have been validated.

7   The National Association of Non-Principals has a sample questionnaire available to download (free of charge for members). (*See* Appendix 1 for details of the website.)

8   Some hospital and community trusts have been using questionnaires developed by their audit departments. Many of these have not been subjected to testing or review and may not give valid or reliable results. Check before use!

You may want to find out what other people in your hospital trust or primary care organisation are using so that co-ordinated surveys can be carried out. If they are, ensure that your own results can be differentiated if you want to use the results for your own development, not just that of the service as a whole.

(iii) Audio or videotape review of consultations

A well-tested way of examining consultation skills is to tape actual consultations (after obtaining consent) and then review them with a checklist. Videotape gives you more information but audiotape can be used in situations where this is not available. A useful checklist for assessing the consultation appears in Tate's book on communication.[7] A suitable consent form is included in that book too, if you do not already use one in your surgery or clinic – if you haven't got one, this might be one of your learning tasks!

You might want to start by reviewing the following five tasks to determine how completely you had achieved them in ten consultations. Look at how well you have:

- established the reason why the patient had come to the surgery or clinic at that time
- defined the problem(s) and made a working diagnosis
- worked out with the patient how serious the problem was, how it could be managed and whether you made an agreed plan for the future
- explained your understanding of the problem to the patient and checked that the explanation was understood and accepted
- used the time to best advantage, concentrated on the main reasons why the patient attended, but utilised suitable opportunities for relevant health advice.

Alternatively, you could use a scale (*see* Box 8.5) to establish what sort of consulting style you use, and whether you vary it according to the needs of the patient.

Box 8.5: Consultation styles

Doctor-centred	*Rating*	*Patient-centred*
I did most of the talking	5 4 3 2 1 1 2 3 4 5	Patient did most of the talking
I asked mostly closed questions	5 4 3 2 1 1 2 3 4 5	I asked mostly open questions
I was mainly interested in problems	5 4 3 2 1 1 2 3 4 5	I was mainly interested in the person
It is my medical agenda that is most important	5 4 3 2 1 1 2 3 4 5	It is the patient's agenda that is most important

continued overleaf

I felt responsible for my patient's problems	5 4 3 2 1 1 2 3 4 5	I felt the patient kept the responsibility
I usually tried to control and guide the consultation	5 4 3 2 1 1 2 3 4 5	I usually let the patient control and guide the consultation
I usually chose the management options and plans	5 4 3 2 1 1 2 3 4 5	The patient usually chose the management options and plans
I believe in telling the patient what is wrong	5 4 3 2 1 1 2 3 4 5	I believe in reaching a shared understanding

In comparison with the above score for this patient, where are you usually?

A doctor-centred consulter	5 4 3 2 1 1 2 3 4 5	A patient-centred consulter

If you only take a few consultations – say, ten – you will need to reflect and record how the variations might have affected your consultation style. For example, you will be much more doctor-centred if the patient has a serious condition – such as a myocardial infarction – than if you are discussing the relative merits of starting on anti-hypertensive treatment with someone with repeated raised blood pressure readings but no risk factors. A larger number of consultations helps you to determine your usual style. You will then need to get some feedback on whether patients or colleagues regard this as satisfactory or if you need to make some changes.

Once you feel able to review your consultations yourself, it would be useful to involve other people in the assessment – perhaps a colleague so that you could review each other's consultations. Always remember the rules of constructive feedback: you comment on your own consultation first, selecting the things you did well, then the things that could be improved, before your colleague does the same. Make factual observations based on the evidence before you – 'I didn't notice that the patient was turning away and wasn't listening at that point', not 'I made a right mess of explaining that'.

You may be using video-recording of your consultations or simulated surgery for assessing your skills as part of the qualifications for the Membership or Fellowship of the Royal College of General Practitioners, so that external review will provide your feedback.

(iv) Seminar review of consultations and reflective feedback

Balint pioneered seminar groups that examine the use of the doctor as treatment. The groups use some of the techniques employed in brief psychoanalytical therapy.[8] The technique has since been used in other fields such as the management of sexual problems.[9] It is particularly helpful if you are having difficulty with the so-called 'heart-sink' or 'fat-file' patients. It is a technique you could utilise to identify your learning needs by exposure to the critique from the group, and to give you an opportunity to reflect on the consultation. You might also use the presentation and discussion in the seminar as a way of meeting your learning needs and improving your consultation skills.

The seminar group is a meeting of peers, of already qualified and experienced medical practitioners, moderated and facilitated by a leader of more experience. The seminar group listens to, interprets and reflects on the work done by the individual doctor in the same way that the doctor works with the patient to formulate a hypothesis about the underlying causes of the problem.

Individual encounters presented to a seminar group can be explored with different interpretations and reflections offered by members of the group. Possible new hypotheses can be put forward and tested with further reflection. This method of working takes forward both our knowledge and our skill gained from the individual patient under discussion and also utilises the understanding for future patients.

The investigation during the consultation is concerned not only with the narrative and physical examination, but also with feelings produced in the doctor and the patient. These feelings in the doctor are a valuable source of information about what feelings the patient might arouse in other people and how these may be produced. The doctor therefore has to be aware of which feelings, arising within him or herself, are produced by the patient and which are his or her own.

You can also carry out this type of reflective examination of the processes of the consultation as a written exercise, either using the processes outlined for the seminar discussion, or as an analysis of the narrative that occurs in the consultation and your contribution to it.[10] You will identify more learning needs from this process if you do it in a group or with feedback from a mentor.

Stage 3: set your priorities and define your learning objectives

Look back at Stage 1 for your standards for relationships with patients. Match your learning needs with one or more of the standards in Box 8.2 or others you have set yourself.

You might want to improve your consultation skills by learning how to cope better with 'heart-sink patients' so that you no longer find them so infuriating. You would also reduce your stress levels and improve your health in the process. Your objective would be 'to be able to demonstrate calmer and more empathetic consultations with "heart-sink patients" by 12 months'.

You could deduce that your doctor-centred consultation style is the result of appointments that are too short, so you will have to learn how to manage the system in a different way to allow for longer and more flexible appointment times. This would also involve your management skills, working with colleagues, and possibly other modules as well. Your objectives would be 'to demonstrate more patient-centred consultations' and 'to show that the patients preferred longer and more flexible appointments'.

You might have established that you are particularly good at written explanations in simple language, but that your verbal explanation skills are not so good because your accent is not always understandable by local people. This might lead you to rewriting some of the information leaflets available, making sure that they were readily available to be printed out quickly. Your objective would be 'to show that well-written and easily accessible leaflets improved patient understanding'.

Stage 4: make an action plan with a timetable

Decide on what method of learning is most appropriate to your task. You may have already identified your preferred learning style – but *see* Chapter 10 for more information.

Good methods for improving consultation skills and relationships with patients are:

- reviewing videotaped consultations with a suitable colleague, mentor or tutor
- seminar groups examining consultation skills
- reviewing significant events involving communication skills
- joint clinics or surgeries with other health professionals
- reflective accounts of the narrative of patient or carer encounters, especially if shared with others
- surveys to obtain feedback on the clarity and usefulness of written or verbal information.

Describe how you will carry out your learning tasks and what you will do by a specified time. Say how your learning will be applied and how and when it will be evaluated. Build in some staging posts so that you do not suddenly get to the end of 12 months and discover that you have only done half of your plan.

You might decide to start with your baseline assessment of how doctor- or patient-centred your consultations were. Then plan to change the appointment system by the end of the next three months. Three months later you assess how doctor- or patient-centred your consultations are, and make any more changes to your style together with advice from a colleague or mentor. Then assess again three months later (i.e. at nine months) and again at the end of 12 months.

The action plan would look like the simple Gantt chart shown in Figure 8.1.

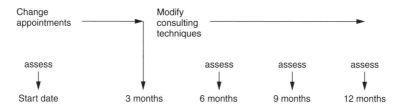

Figure 8.1:   A Gantt chart for your action plan – relationships with patients.

Stage 5: evaluate your progress

You might choose to evaluate and determine the outcomes of your efforts by repeating the learning needs assessment with which you started. If you used a validated patient satisfaction questionnaire then you can compare the results directly. Do not get despondent if only a small change is demonstrated. Change often takes time to become evident, especially if you have also had to alter other parameters such as length of appointments, or who sees patients for what.

Instead of an objective measurement, you might go for a qualitative one. You might value the changes by the degree by which your level of stress or dissatisfaction has been reduced. You might value the feedback from colleagues about your improved skills. You might record the tokens of appreciation from patients and relatives!

EXAMPLE DIARY SHEETS FOR THIS SECTION

Diary sheet for section on relationships with patients EXAMPLE 1	
Stage 1: criteria and outcomes selected	To show that this doctor: 1 treats patients with courtesy and consideration 2 maintains the patient's dignity, especially during physical examination 3 informs patients and carers about their condition in a way that they can understand 4 empowers patients to take decisions about their management 5 keeps information about patients confidential, explains the necessity to others and seeks consent before sharing information; consults or discusses patients where confidential information cannot be overheard.
Stage 2: methods of assessment	1 DIALOGUE consultation satisfaction questionnaire analysis of personal consultations. 2 Review two sessions of videotaped consultations with your tutor. 3 Audit of enquiries from outside bodies for patient information to determine compliance with the guidelines for confidentiality. 4 Audit of management of enquiries about results by patients or others for confidentiality.
Stage 3: which objectives have been selected for action this year and why	1 Criteria 1 and 2 came out as well regarded by patients; little improvement needed so not high priority. 2 Criterion 3 needs improvement and fits in with the need for readily available information sheets identified from needs assessment in the modules 'good medical practice', 'training' and 'relationships with colleagues'. 3 Criterion 4 did not seem well met and might be due to insufficient information – so put criterion 3 higher.

Diary sheet for section on relationships with patients EXAMPLE 1 *Continued*	
	4 Audit of enquiries from outside bodies met the standard set, but a problem was identified with individuals. No check on the identity of phone enquiries was made, so a change in guidelines was needed. The objectives selected are to: • improve the quality of verbal and written information • incorporate a check on the identity of phone callers asking for patient information.
Stage 4: the action plan	Baseline assessment as above. By 3 months: obtain, read and modify if necessary written patient information sheets on cardiovascular disease and obesity.[11,12] Add advice on phone enquiries to the guidelines on enquiries for patient information. By 6 months: use the leaflets in the consultation for verbal explanations and to give to patients; give simple feedback questionnaire with leaflet for patient evaluation. At 9 months: continue the above; start analysis of feedback comments. At 12 months: reapply assessment; finish analysis of feedback.
Stage 5: evaluation of progress and dissemination	1 Feedback from simple questionnaire of understanding and helpfulness of the information received. 2 Review of changes in consultation skills and patient satisfaction. 3 Written information materials made easily accessible to colleagues. 4 Adherence to guidelines for phone enquiries shows understanding of the hazards.

Diary sheet for section on relationships with patients EXAMPLE 2	
Stage 1: criteria and outcomes selected	To show that this doctor: 1 obtains informed consent to physical examination, investigations and treatment 2 keeps information about patients confidential, explains the necessity to others and seeks consent before sharing information; consults or discusses patients where confidential information cannot be overheard.[13]
Stage 2: methods of assessment	1 DISQ satisfaction questionnaire analysis of personal consultations. 2 Review four clinics that have been audiotaped. 3 Keep a record of all enquiries for information about patients for one week and how they were handled.
Stage 3: which objectives have been selected for action this year and why	1 Giving information about the reasons for physical examinations needs improvement. 2 Patients do not understand why investigations are being done. 3 Information and understanding about treatment are at a higher level of performance. 4 Information about patients is often passed on in public places where others can overhear. The objectives selected are to: • improve the quality of verbal and written information about physical examination and investigations • arrange to give information to colleagues in a clinical or clerical room without other people not involved in the care of the patient being present.

Diary sheet for section on relationships with patients
EXAMPLE 2 *Continued*

Stage 4: the action plan	Baseline assessment as above. By 3 months: write and pilot information on common reasons for physical examination and investigations and what they entail. By 6 months: send out the leaflets with the appointment; ask the patients if they have any queries when they attend; use a feedback questionnaire for patient evaluation. At 9 months: continue the above; start analysis of feedback comments. At 12 months: reapply assessment; finish analysis of feedback.
Stage 5: evaluation of progress	1　Feedback from simple questionnaire of understanding and helpfulness of the information received. 2　Review of changes in consultation skills and patient satisfaction. 3　Results disseminated to colleagues. 4　Written information materials made accessible to colleagues. 5　Colleagues and staff understand the need for private exchange of information about patients.

Diary sheet for section on relationships with patients
EXAMPLE 3

Stage 1: criteria and outcomes selected	To show that this doctor: 1 apologises appropriately when things go wrong, and has an adequate complaints procedure in place 2 can justify why ending a professional relationship with a patient is fair and can communicate those reasons to the patient.
Stage 2: methods of assessment	1 Review of complaints and feedback from patients. 2 Review of staff assessments. 3 Review with practice team of removal of patients from practice list, recording reasons and methods of communication of removal.
Stage 3: which objectives have been selected for action this year and why	1 Identified need for more speedy personal response when responding to complaints to reduce patient frustration and doctor fear and anger. 2 Identified need to learn better skills in communicating after personally committing errors. 3 Justification seems adequately covered, but communication of those reasons to patients is inadequate. The objectives selected are to: • set a target to write a personal initial response to complaints within 48 hours, and to review the initial response to reply within 72 hours • show greater skills in apologising for errors • improve letters to patients advising them of the reasons for removal from the practice list.
Stage 4: the action plan	Baseline assessment as above. By 3 months: the response to any complaint received is to meet the time targets. Attend a course in assertiveness training to learn how to apologise without feeling or being defensive. Obtain examples of letters advising patients of removal from list and adapt for practice use. By 6 months: review progress. At 9 months: review progress. At 12 months: reapply assessment.
Stage 5: evaluation of progress	1 Review repeat assessments for progress. 2 Discuss with practice team. 3 Advise primary care organisation (PCO) of revised complaints procedures.

References

1 Wakley G, Chambers R and Dieppe P (2001) *Musculoskeletal Matters in Primary Care*. Radcliffe Medical Press, Oxford.

2 Royal Pharmaceutical Society of Great Britain (1997) *From Compliance to Concordance: towards shared goals in medicine taking.* Royal Pharmaceutical Society of Great Britain, London.

3 General Medical Council (2001) *Good Medical Practice*. General Medical Council, London.

4 Howie JGR, Heaney D, Maxwell M and Walker JJ (1998) A comparison of the Patient Enablement Instrument (PEI) against two established satisfaction scales as an outcome measure of primary care consultations. *Family Practice.* **15**: 165–71.

5 Grogan S, Conner M, Norman P *et al.* (2000) Validation of a questionnaire measuring patient satisfaction with general practitioner services. *Quality in Health Care.* **9**: 210–15.

6 Steine S, Finset A and Laerum E (2001) A new, brief, questionnaire (PEF) developed in primary care for measuring patients' experience of interaction, emotion and consultation outcome. *Family Practice.* **18**: 410–18.

7 Tate P (2003) *The Doctor's Communication Handbook* (4e). Radcliffe Medical Press, Oxford.

8 Balint M (1964) *The Doctor, His Patient and the Illness*. Pitman, London.

9 Skrine R and Montford H (2001) *Psychosexual Medicine: an introduction*. Arnold, London.

10 Shapiro J and Ross V (2002) Application of narrative theory and therapy to the practice of family medicine. *Family Medicine.* **34**: 96–100.

11 Chambers R, Wakley G and Iqbal Z (2001) *Cardiovascular Disease Matters in Primary Care*. Radcliffe Medical Press, Oxford.

12 Chambers R and Wakley G (2002) *Obesity and Overweight Matters in Primary Care*. Radcliffe Medical Press, Oxford.

13 General Medical Council (2001) *Confidentiality: protecting and providing information*. General Medical Council, London.

9

Working with colleagues

Introduction

Teams produce better patient care than single practitioners operating in a fragmented way.[1] Effective teams make the most of the different contributions from individuals in various clinical disciplines in delivering patient care. The characteristics of effective teams are:

- sharing aims
- having a clear understanding of the contributions each discipline makes
- establishing good and free communication between team members
- ensuring that team members can enhance their skills.

A team approach helps different team members adopt a reasoned or evidence-based approach to patient care. Each member has to be able to justify his or her approach to the rest of the team.

The future shape of healthcare delivery centres on teamwork because:

- the traditional boundaries between primary and secondary care are disappearing
- care is more integrated
- access to primary care is diversifying
- an increased range of healthcare services will be provided at primary care level
- the primary care workforce is increasingly multidisciplinary
- nurses are developing extended skills and responsibilities
- health and social services planning and provision will become integrated.

Clinical governance will be practised at a service level through multi-disciplinary teams working across agencies.[2] Teams which encourage participation are more likely to achieve a patient-centred service, work together as a team and be more efficient.

Good communication is essential for good teamwork. You need:

- regular staff meetings – which managers and staff endeavour to attend
- demonstration that decisions taken at meetings are implemented

- a fail-safe system for passing on important messages
- a way to share news so that everyone is notified accurately of changes as soon as the information is available
- opportunities for quieter members of the team to contribute
- feedback given and received about your role in the team
- everyone to feel that they are part of, and believe in, the decision making.

Team-building starts from the top. Managers and senior clinicians should set good examples that encourage trust and respect from other colleagues. Without this, no organisation will be able to function at its full potential. This takes time, effort and consistency but you'll reap the rewards.

Clinical teams

Integrated nursing teams have existed for years but interdisciplinary teams require more development.[3] In a clinical team where members may have overlapping clinical responsibilities, make clear and unambiguous handover arrangements. Select the leader of the team for his or her leadership skills rather than on the basis of status, hierarchy or availability. Include all the relevant professions serving a practice population in the membership of the team. Include nurses, doctors, paramedics, pharmacists, therapists and other operational staff and clinical leads in clinical improvement teams.

Teamwork does not necessarily follow just because professionals are working alongside one another or contributing to the same patient management decisions. The nature of the professional structure, as well as historical and attitudinal barriers, can and do contribute to difficulties which inhibit teamwork. Problems can arise from competing demands, diverse lines of management, poor communication and personality factors. Status and gender effects are particularly noticeable in the health service!

A number of other issues are likely to make an impact on teamworking. The changing health and social environment, new government policies, and professional and technological developments produce a rapidly changing background to the establishment of working teams.

Think how you can involve the public in your decisions.[4] Recognise and include the patient, carer or representative as an essential member of the healthcare team at individual patient-centred team level or at practice level. Giving patients power to make informed decisions about their well-being, health and social care will require a more sophisticated approach to teamworking to meet patients' needs and expectations.

Ensure that the sharing of patient information within the team is in accordance with current confidentiality requirements.

How will you demonstrate satisfactory standards?

Remind yourself of the stages of the learning cycle for appraisal (*see* Figure A).

Stage 1: setting standards and outcomes

Look at the following criteria for a good doctor working with colleagues listed in Box 9.1. They are derived from *Good Medical Practice* – standards set

---

Box 9.1: Criteria for working with colleagues

You should:

1 treat your colleagues fairly – do not discriminate against colleagues, including those applying for posts, on the grounds of sex, race, or disability
2 not allow your personal opinions about your colleagues' lifestyle, culture, beliefs, race, gender, sexuality or age to affect your professional relationship
3 resist the temptation to appear superior by denigrating the care patients have received from others
4 respect the skills and contributions of your colleagues
5 maintain professional relationships with patients and ensure that informed consent is obtained to sharing information necessary for their care by the team
6 keep open lines of communication with colleagues both within and outside your team
7 make sure that others understand your professional status and specialty, what roles and responsibilities you have and who is responsible for each aspect of the patient's care
8 join in with reviews and audits of the standards and performance of the team, and with any steps necessary to remedy deficiencies
9 be supportive of other team members when there are difficulties with health, conduct or performance
10 have satisfactory arrangements for handing over responsibility for patients, both for communicating information and for the quality of the care they will receive, when you are not available to provide it
11 make suitable arrangements for the referral of patients to a healthcare professional of known competence or accountability to provide additional facilities or care.

You may need to take a role as a leader of a team with additional responsibilities for ensuring that others also carry out the criteria above. As a leader you have the responsibility for making sure that standards are met and problems are tackled.

---

by the General Medical Council.[5] You may want to add some others as well or expand the details given in the box.

Stage 2: identify your learning needs

You may decide to incorporate your learning needs assessment for working with colleagues together with one of the other areas, so that you cover more than one in a single assessment. For this type of combined assessment, you might use:

- patient feedback or patient satisfaction surveys (*see* Chapter 8)
- audio, videotape or seminar review of consultations (*see* Chapter 8)
- audit of protocols and guidelines (*see* Chapter 12) for checking how well confidentiality or referral procedures are followed
- self-assessment (*see* Chapter 6) using a rating scale to assess your skills and attitudes in consultation
- reflective practice identifying your learning needs or patients' needs (*see* Chapter 6)
- evaluation of consent issues (*see* Chapter 11) to look at how you deal with or pass on information to others
- examination of patients' records (*see* Chapter 13) to determine how patient care is managed by the team and other agencies
- patient complaint reviews (*see* Chapter 12) to identify the communication problems that have led to a complaint being made.

Learning needs assessment techniques that are particularly suitable for use in determining standards for working with colleagues are:

- significant event audit
- constructive feedback with peer observation
- 360° feedback
- role description
- identifying team difficulties.

These five methods are considered in more detail below.

(i) Significant event audit

Significant event auditing is a structured approach to reviewing events that have occurred. The examination of case histories of selected patients provides a rich source of material for learning. While all significant events have the capacity to identify areas requiring improvement, most will demonstrate adequate standards of care.

To carry out a significant event audit, a group of people involved in that event should meet together. They should agree on a review of the event with a no-blame attitude and mutual trust and respect for each other. Confidentiality rules must be set out right from the start. If the patient or the participants in the care of the patient are identifiable (and they usually are) then all must agree on confidentiality about what is discussed and any reporting must be anonymised. The members of the group discuss the events and some or all of the following:

- the management of the event
- any opportunities for prevention
- the follow-up
- the implications for the patient, the relatives and the community
- the actions of the clinical and non-clinical members of the team
- what action should be taken as a result of the review
- how the actions (if required) will be evaluated or monitored.

Some significant events are adverse incidents. These are events where something has clearly gone wrong, and there is a need to establish what happened, what was preventable and what changes are needed. Some adverse incidents reveal only minor risks or ones that would occur extremely infrequently and these will be judged by the team as not requiring any changes.

Box 9.2:

A street party was organised to celebrate the Queen's Jubilee. Unfortunately a barbecue was placed too near the wooden rail of the ramp leading up to the surgery entrance and it caught fire. It was felt unlikely that such an incident would recur, so the wooden handrail was replaced with another, rather than changing the design to a more expensive one that was not flammable.

By contrast, an adverse event that is very serious, however rare, may require action.

Box 9.3:

Dr Little was injured by a psychotic patient who attacked her with an axe hidden in his coat. A review of the panic button position and response arrangements prompted changes in the arrangements for such emergencies.

In hospital settings, a range of confidential reviews, such as those in maternity events, deaths and suicides, provide useful occasions to review the role of teamworking and other issues.

Risk management reporting of adverse events and near misses should be part of routine clinical governance management. In risk management reporting there should be an easily identifiable route for action that should include:

- identifying and recording the adverse incident or near miss
- reporting to an overall monitoring body in the workplace or organisation
- analysis of the incident
- grouping together any similar occurrences to determine any trends
- discussing any necessary changes with the people involved
- implementing any changes necessary.

A group of colleagues and staff who review events together allow shared analysis and implementation of any necessary changes. Significant event audit uses teamworking to highlight any problems with the relationships between colleagues and staff and to provide agreed solutions that can be implemented.

(ii) Constructive feedback with peer observation

Your effectiveness depends, for a large part, on how you function within a team. Obtaining direct feedback from the administrative and clinical members, as well as from your peers, can be quite scary and is often resisted by both sides. It is sometimes easier to receive such feedback if it is structured to include some items that can be praised as well as some criticism. An assessment rating form such as the one in Box 9.4 can be used. Initially people are often only willing to complete such a form anonymously but, with increasing confidence in

---

Box 9.4:   Assessment form for colleagues and staff

Name of person being assessed: Dr......................................

He/she is polite and courteous	Always	Usually	Sometimes	Never
He/she is professional in his/her manner	Always	Usually	Sometimes	Never
He/she is co-operative in accepting necessary extra duties	Always	Usually	Sometimes	Never
He/she is punctual and keeps to time	Always	Usually	Sometimes	Never
He/she seeks advice and help readily	Always	Usually	Sometimes	Never
He/she accepts criticism constructively	Always	Usually	Sometimes	Never
He/she appreciates my role and skills	Always	Usually	Sometimes	Never
He/she works in an organised manner	Always	Usually	Sometimes	Never
Patients make complimentary remarks about him/her	Always	Usually	Sometimes	Never
Patients make critical remarks to me about him/her	Always	Usually	Sometimes	Never
He/she is easy to get on with	Always	Usually	Sometimes	Never
He/she fits in well with the team	Always	Usually	Sometimes	Never

seeing how the form is used, a more open approach can be made. Any comments recorded should always be factual and about what is done or not done, and should not be comments on people's personal characteristics.

(iii) 360° feedback

This collects together perceptions from a number of different participants, as seen in Figure 9.1.

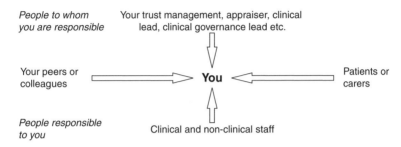

Figure 9.1:   360° feedback.

The wider the spread of people giving feedback, the more rounded the picture. Each individual gives a feedback questionnaire to at least three people in each of the groups in Figure 9.1. An independent person then collects and collates the questionnaires and discusses the results with the individual. A computerised version called *Insight* is available from Edgecumbe Consulting (*see* Appendix 1). The main disadvantage of this method is that it can sometimes be spoilt by malicious comments against which individuals cannot readily defend themselves.

(iv) Role description

We often think that we know what are the roles, expertise and responsibilities of other people who work with us. However, it is also clear that we often make assumptions that can lead to poorer management of the patient.

Perhaps, too, other members of your team do not know what your areas of expertise are. If you are qualified in, and enthusiastic about, minor surgery, you may be annoyed to find that patients are waiting to be seen at a hospital clinic when you could do the necessary treatment at the surgery. If you are a specialist in elderly person care, but have a lot of experience in diabetic care, you will be irritated if another health professional refers a patient to the endocrinologist for 'sorting out'.

Make a written list of your roles, expertise and responsibilities and record those of your colleagues in a loose-leaf folder (for easy updating as staff changes

---

Box 9.5:

Dr Dash visited a patient with axillary vein thrombosis at home. The patient looked after her elderly mother who had senile dementia and had been very unsettled by her daughter's admission to hospital. The doctor readily agreed that it would be best if the patient had home monitoring of her anticoagulation treatment. He left a message for the district nurse to call to do this. He was dismayed to receive a call from the patient two weeks later to ask why no-one had been. On enquiry he found that the district nurse covering the area in which the patient lived did not regard this as part of her duties and had notified the hospital clinic of this, not the GP. The hospital clinic had sent the patient an appointment which she had cancelled, believing that alternative arrangements had been made.

---

occur). Identify the gaps in your knowledge and the gaps in the provision of services or expertise available to patients.

(v) Identifying team difficulties

The book *What Stress in Primary Care!* looks at many situations where you might identify difficulties in the practice or workplace team.[6] The checklist in Box 9.6 might show that you need to learn more about how to look after your colleagues.

Box 9.6:   Checklist for care and support of staff in the workplace

If a member of staff or colleague is tearful and upset, does someone enquire what is wrong and offer to support him or her?	Always Usually Seldom Never
If someone is off sick for several months, will he or she be able to start back on reduced hours of work or with added support?	Always Usually Seldom Never
Would an applicant who is normally in a wheelchair, or who wears a hearing aid, be considered equally to someone without these disabilities for an advertised post?	Always Usually Seldom Never
Are staff and colleagues registered with doctors who are independent of their workplace?	Always Usually Seldom Never
Is there gossip about people's personal problems?	Always Usually Seldom Never

continued opposite

If someone came to work appearing to have a drug or alcohol problem on several occasions, would someone tackle him or her about it?	Always Usually Seldom Never
Is there flexibility to change working hours if someone has problems at home?	Always Usually Seldom Never
Are there recognised avenues for staff and colleagues to vent their concerns and worries?	Always Usually Seldom Never

If the answers to the checklist are mainly 'seldom' or 'never', your team needs to co-operate to make changes. If you are the leader of the team, it is your responsibility to make sure the changes happen.

Stage 3: set your priorities and define your learning objectives

Look back at Stage 1 at your standards for working with colleagues. Match your learning needs with one or more of the criteria in Box 9.1 or others you have set yourself.

You might have identified that the roles and responsibilities of individuals in the patient management team are poorly understood. The objective might be to provide a folder with a summary page for each team member describing relevant roles and responsibilities.

A review may have shown that support of staff who are having personal or work difficulties has been neglected. As a team leader you need to put in place some procedures to remedy the situation. Your objective might be to provide each member of staff with a named person inside the workplace and a contact outside the workplace who would be responsible for providing that individual with support.

An audit of your arrangements for referral of patients may show unacceptable referrals to persons of unknown competence or accountability such as alternative practitioners. Your objective would be to have a list of alternative practitioners with their professional qualifications and regulatory bodies recorded for reference in your workplace.

A significant event audit may reveal that communication with the out-of-hours cover by doctors failed several times during the interval between the end of surgery consultations and the takeover by the deputising co-operative.

The objective would be to provide the doctor on call with a dedicated mobile phone and ensure that all team members had a record of that number.

Stage 4: make an action plan with a timetable

Decide what method of learning is most appropriate to your task. You may have already identified your preferred learning style – but *see* Chapter 10 for more information.

Good ways of improving your skills of working with colleagues are:

- ensuring that you know who are the individuals included in your work-place team
- arranging to meet formally and informally with other members of the team
- keeping a record of how to contact other team members
- knowing who does what and how well
- making sure that team members have the necessary knowledge, skills and attitudes before delegating responsibilities to them
- encouraging team members to develop skills, acquire knowledge and take responsibility
- behaving politely and courteously and apologising if you do not when under stress
- keeping records that can be understood (and read) by other members of the team for good continuity of care
- keeping information confidential unless there is a need to know and con-sent for the transfer of information
- avoiding behaviour that could be regarded as bullying, denigrating or harassing.

Describe how you will carry out your learning tasks and what you will do by a specified time. Say how your learning will be applied and how and when it will be evaluated. Build in some staging posts so that you do not suddenly get to the end of 12 months and discover that you have only completed half of your plan.

A simple Gantt chart like the one in Figure 9.2 helps you to track what you are going to do and when.

Stage 5: evaluate your progress

You might choose to evaluate and determine the outcome of your efforts by repeating the learning needs assessment that you started with. You might value the feedback from colleagues about your improved skills or attitudes.

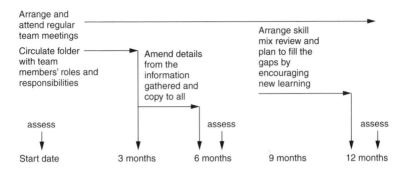

Figure 9.2:   A Gantt chart for your action plan – working with colleagues.

Significant event audit might show the degree to which changes made have influenced teamworking. You might find that the checklist of support for staff shows considerable improvement, but that a complaint from a patient has caused even more stress! You might evaluate the changes by the degree to which your own level of stress or dissatisfaction has been reduced.

References

1   Wakley G, Chambers R and Field S (2000) *Continuing Professional Development in Primary Care: making it happen.* Radcliffe Medical Press, Oxford.

2   Chambers R and Wakley G (2000) *Making Clinical Governance Work for You.* Radcliffe Medical Press, Oxford.

3   Elwyn G and Smail J (1998) *Integrated Teams in Primary Care.* Radcliffe Medical Press, Oxford.

4   Chambers R (2000) *Involving Patients and the Public.* Radcliffe Medical Press, Oxford.

5   General Medical Council (2001) *Good Medical Practice.* General Medical Council, London.

6   Chambers R and Davies M (1999) *What Stress in Primary Care!* Royal College of General Practitioners, London.

EXAMPLE DIARY SHEETS FOR THIS SECTION

Diary sheet for section on working with colleagues EXAMPLE 1	
Stage 1: criteria and outcomes selected	To show that this doctor: 1 has satisfactory arrangements for handing over responsibility for patients, both for communicating information and for the quality of the care they will receive, when he or she is not available to provide it 2 makes suitable arrangements for the referral of patients to a healthcare professional of known competence or accountability to provide additional facilities or care.
Stage 2: methods of assessment	1 Significant event monitoring. 2 Role description.
Stage 3: which objectives have been selected for action this year and why	These parameters were found to be poor so the objectives are to: • demonstrate that communication between doctors and district nurses has improved • acquire and record knowledge of roles and responsibilities of allied health professionals (AHPs).
Stage 4: the action plan	Baseline assessment as above. By 3 months: arrangements to visit AHPs over the 12 month period. Meeting with district nurse representatives to discuss lines of communication. By 6 months: piloting of central message-taker for district nurses and supply of all contact telephone numbers to wards, practices and central message centre, funded from existing clerical budget. At 9 months: completion of visits to AHPs; personal resource file completed. At 12 months: reapply assessment, feedback results.
Stage 5: evaluation of progress	1 AHPs happy to meet and communication as well as knowledge improved; visits arranged to spread over the 12 months to avoid overload of work. 2 Feedback from users of central message-taker for district nurses suggested system worked well. 3 Assessment showed improved communication and knowledge of each other's roles and responsibilities and better understanding of patients' needs.

Diary sheet for section on working with colleagues EXAMPLE 2	
Stage 1: criteria and outcomes selected	To show that this doctor: 1 does not allow personal opinions about colleagues to affect professional relationships 2 does not denigrate the care patients have received from others.
Stage 2: methods of assessment	1 Significant event audit. 2 360° feedback. 3 Identifying team difficulties. 4 Patient complaint.
Stage 3: which objectives have been selected for action this year and why	1 Feedback from some colleagues suggests that my attitudes are sometimes abrupt and appear uncaring towards colleagues in difficulty. 2 A complaint from a patient accused a colleague of deficiencies of care after interpreting comments made by me as criticism of that colleague. The objectives are to: • reduce my stress levels • change my communications with colleagues for the better • improve my communication skills with patients.
Stage 4: the action plan	Baseline assessment as above. By 3 months: finish assessment of sources of stress. By 6 months: put in place increased consultation intervals with breaks for refreshment and meeting with colleagues. At 9 months: review stress levels at the end of each working day. At 12 months: reapply assessment, analyse feedback.
Stage 5: evaluation of progress	1 Examination of causes of the communication difficulties reveals high stress levels and inadequate breaks in the working day. 2 Negotiation of different working pattern relieves the stress to some degree and allows time for communication with colleagues. 3 A better understanding of colleagues' working patterns and difficulties established.

10

Teaching and training

Introduction

Doctors with special interests or responsibilities for teaching and training – of students, junior staff, colleagues or patients – may weight the time and effort they spend on their personal and professional development and collecting evidence for their appraisal portfolio towards addressing this section. Doctors who combine a part-time post as a teacher and trainer with clinical practice will produce a more substantial body of evidence about their teaching practice as opposed to doctors whose teaching is an incidental part of their daily job.

You may demonstrate how you have become more knowledgeable, skilled and proficient as an educationalist and how you are able to apply your work over a variety of clinical educational situations and settings.

Being a competent teacher requires practice and continual improvement so that you should:[1]

- stimulate the learner
- interest and involve the learner
- prepare well so that the context and content is clear and focused
- encourage the learner – with positive feedback
- understand the learner's needs
- have an appropriate plan to meet the learner's needs
- use a style of delivery that suits the learner's needs
- evaluate the teaching and the learning
- refine future teaching in light of evaluation
- be a lifelong learner.

This section of *Good Medical Practice* covers 'appraising and assessing' as well as 'teaching and training'.[2] Remind yourself of the definition of appraisal we gave in Chapter 1: '**Appraisal** is an official or formal evaluation of the strengths and weaknesses of someone or something' (*Collins COBUILD English Dictionary,* 1999). **Assessment** is a way of measuring a learner's achievements, normally after they have worked through a learning programme of one sort or another.

It has a 'pass' and 'fail' standard. An assessment should be:

- valid – it measures what it is supposed to measure (in the objective already agreed)
- reliable – it measures with essentially the same result each time
- practicable – it is easy to do in terms of cost, time and skills of the assessors
- fair to the learners and the teachers
- useful to the learners and the teachers
- acceptable – in terms of cultural and gender issues
- appropriate – to what has been taught and learnt on the programme.[2]

Competence is a person's ability to perform; their competencies are their total capability (what they can do, not necessarily what they do). An appropriate definition of 'competence' is 'the state of having the knowledge, judgement, skills, energy, experience and motivation required to respond adequately to the demands of one's professional responsibilities'.[3]

Regarding **learning styles**, there is a lot of evidence to suggest that different individuals learn in different ways. Learners have preferences for certain kinds of information and ways of using that information to learn. Several models have been described. No one model is the 'correct' one.[1]

1 *Convergent and divergent thinkers*: convergent thinkers tend to find a single solution to a problem set to them, whereas divergent thinkers tend to generate new ideas, expand ideas and explore widely.
2 *Serialists and holists*: serialists learn best by going one step at a time, whereas holists learn best by getting the big picture at the start and then filling in the steps.
3 *Deep and surface processors*: deep processors like to get at the main points of an article in order to understand it, whereas surface processors like to read through the material, remembering as much as possible.

Honey and Mumford have done an enormous amount of detailed work on learning styles.[4] They describe four different basic styles, which are described below. Many individuals are a combination of two styles while others are fairly well rounded and possess features of all four styles in similar proportions; some people are very much of one style only.

- *Activists* like to be fully involved in new experiences, are open-minded, will try anything once, and thrive on the challenge of new experiences but soon get bored, wanting to go on to the next challenge. They are gregarious and like to be the centre of attention. Activists learn best with new experiences, short activities, situations where they can be centre stage (chairing meetings, leading discussions), and when allowed to generate new ideas, have a go at things or brainstorm ideas.
- *Reflectors* like to stand back, think about things thoroughly and collect a lot of information before coming to a conclusion. They are cautious, take

a back seat in meetings and discussions, adopt a low profile and appear tolerant and unruffled. When they do act, it is by using the wide picture of their own and others' views. Reflectors learn best from situations where they are allowed to watch and think about activities, think before acting, carry out research first of all, review evidence, produce carefully constructed reports and reach decisions in their own time.

- *Theorists* like to adapt and integrate observations into logical maps and models, using step-by-step processes. They tend to be perfectionists, detached, analytical and objective and reject anything that is subjective, flippant and lateral thinking in nature. Theorists learn best from activities where there are plans, maps and models to describe what is going on, time to explore the methodology, structured situations with a clear purpose, and when offered complex situations to understand and they are intellectually stretched.
- *Pragmatists* like to try out ideas, theories and techniques to see if they work in practice. They will act quickly and confidently on ideas that attract them and are impatient with ruminating and open-ended discussions. They are down-to-earth people who like solving problems and making practical decisions, responding to problems as a challenge. Pragmatists learn best when there is an obvious link between the subject and their jobs. They enjoy trying out techniques with coaching and feedback, practical issues, real problems to solve and when given the immediate chance to implement what has been learned.

In practical terms, you need to tailor your teaching and training to the learners' individual needs.

How will you demonstrate satisfactory standards?

Remind yourself of the stages of the learning cycle for appraisal (*see* Figure A).

Stage 1: setting standards and outcomes

Look at the following criteria for teaching and training, appraising and assessing, listed in Box 10.1. They are derived from *Good Medical Practice*.[2] You may want to add some others as well or expand the details given in the box. These describe the criteria you will be showing that you meet in this section of the appraisal paperwork.

Box 10.1: Criteria for teaching and training, appraising and assessing

You should:

1 be honest and objective when appraising or assessing the performance of any doctor, including those you have supervised or trained
2 provide honest and justifiable comments when giving references for, or writing reports about, colleagues; these will include all relevant information about their competence, performance and conduct
3 contribute to the education of students or colleagues willingly
4 develop the skills, attitudes and practices of a competent teacher if you have responsibilities for teaching
5 ensure that students and junior colleagues are properly supervised in line with the responsibilities you have for teaching them.

Stage 2: identify your learning needs

Choose your methods of identifying your learning needs to determine how standards of your own practice compare with the criteria given in *Good Medical Practice*.

You could:

- collate evidence of your own performance as an educationalist as compared with other standards (this will include seeking feedback from others).
- undertake a review of your learning style and/or that of those whom you teach.

These two methods are described in more detail below.

(i) Collate evidence of your own performance as an educationalist as compared with other standards

Facilitators appointed to the Accredited Professional Development (APD) of the Royal College of General Practitioners demonstrate their competence in eight main areas.[5,6] These are adapted and abbreviated below. You will need to seek feedback from students and colleagues whom you teach or train, appraise or assess, about how you fare in any or all of these competency areas.

1 Competency area: understands the healthcare context and can make realistic allowances for potential problems while assisting problem-solving.
   - Understands health context.
     A competent educationalist will be familiar with the primary or secondary care setting. He or she will be able to talk and respond

knowledgeably about the competing demands within a learner's everyday work.
- Problem-solving.
  Can show examples of effective problem-solving and facilitation of change that will assist learners to overcome contextual barriers.
2 Competency area: understands the potential for conflicts of interest to arise.
- Understands the potential for conflicts of interest to arise between educationalist and learner.
  A competent educationalist recognises where the boundaries lie between being an educationalist and other roles such as mentor, pastoral supporter or advocate.
- Understands when patient safety is threatened and how to act accordingly.
  He or she understands when patient safety is threatened and is prepared to take appropriate action in accordance with the BMA's code of ethics.
- Understands the potential for conflicts of interest to arise between the learner and the wider NHS.
  A competent educationalist is familiar with the different perspectives and priorities of an individual practitioner and the team in their work setting, and the wider NHS within the trust or NHS as a whole.
3 Competency area: understands the national priorities and the NHS approach to performance and how this is relevant to the learner's circumstances.
- Understands NHS approach to performance.
  A competent educationalist is familiar with the components of the NHS performance assessment framework (health improvement, fair access, efficiency, effective delivery of appropriate care, user/carer experience, health outcomes).
- Familiar with NHS priorities.
  A competent educationalist is sufficiently familiar with the various clinical and non-clinical priorities of the NHS, at national and relevant local levels, to be able to inform the learner's prioritisation of his or her learning needs.
4 Competency area: understands and practises the principles of adult education.
- Guiding individuals to identify their own personal and professional learning needs in relation to service development needs.
  A competent educationalist will be practised in a variety of techniques for identifying such needs and will know which ones are appropriate for different situations and purposes.
- Setting educational objectives.

A competent educationalist will be able to guide a learner in establishing objectives for the learning plan that are appropriate to his or her personal and professional needs in relation to service development.

- Making a relevant learning plan that relates to the learner's professional practice and ongoing experiences.

    A competent educationalist will review the factors in the past year and beyond that have contributed to the recent performance of the learner, and encourage him or her to set new development objectives for the coming year that are appropriate for the learner and the working context, while identifying the new knowledge, skills and attitudes and additional resources/support that the learner will need.

- Evaluating a relevant learning plan.

    A competent educationalist will know of at least two methods to evaluate learning and be able to guide the learner in the selection of a suitable method of evaluation.

- Motivation to perform well.

    A competent educationalist is able to motivate the learner in relation to continuing quality improvement of all aspects of his or her practice.

- Good feedback.

    A competent educationalist will know of at least one standard model of giving feedback, and its strengths and weaknesses in different situations.

5   Competency area: understands and practises skills in interpersonal working and communication.

- Interpersonal working.

    A competent educationalist will have insight into the drivers and barriers to good interpersonal working. He/she will be able to create a good working relationship with any learner whatever their background, nature or character.

- Communication.

    A competent educationalist will understand what factors contribute to good communication, and what factors interfere with communication. He or she will be able to communicate well with the learner to encourage self-directed learning, to realise strengths and weaknesses in respect of performance at work and with the educational plan. A competent educationalist is non-judgemental, generous in his or her praise, able to listen and hear in a positive manner, is skilled in communicating well in a systematic way, able to establish a rapport with learners whatever their backgrounds and able to reach consensus with the learner about his or her action plan through discussion.

6 Competency area: understands and practises skills in undertaking peer review/appraisal.
   - Arranging the peer review/appraisal meeting.
     A competent educationalist will arrange the peer review/appraisal at a time and place such that there is privacy and protected time.
   - Perform the process of a peer review/appraisal.
     A competent educationalist will set out the objectives of an educational peer review/appraisal, establishing an open and honest discussion, and empowering the individual being reviewed. He or she will base the annual peer review on an in-depth discussion of the learner's portfolio and help the learner redetermine outstanding learning needs in keeping with the points raised above. He or she will create a climate of education and development rather than one that is adversarial or blaming.
   - Definition of appraisal (e.g. Department of Health toolkit at www.appraisals.nhs.uk).
     A competent educationalist will understand that the scope and purpose of appraisal includes: a formal review and planning process taking place at planned intervals (e.g. annual) to understand the factors that have contributed to past performance in order to celebrate good performance and identify ways to improve future performance. He or she will be able to explain the scope and purpose to the person being appraised.
7 Competency area: understands the structure and process of the appraisal, and can help the learner to navigate through the appraisal process.
   - Facilitation of learning programme.
     A competent educationalist can recognise and acknowledge whether the learning that has occurred since the previous appraisal has addressed the learner's needs and fulfilled the GMC's requirements for revalidation. The educationalist will be familiar with the criteria for the duties and responsibilities of doctors as described in a current edition of *Good Medical Practice*.
8 Competency area: understands the standards of information and evidence expected in an appraisal portfolio.
   - Can demonstrate standards of information and evidence.
     A competent educationalist can differentiate between those doctors who submit an appropriate standard of information and evidence about their practice and those who do not; he or she understands what it means for appraisal to be a formative process; he or she understands the meaning of assessment and can make sound judgements about the extent to which work submitted is at least at a 'pass' level – when appraisal and assessment are appropriate.

(ii) Ascertaining learning styles – both yours and the match between the way you teach and train and others' learning styles

The learning styles questionnaire devised by Honey and Mumford is an 80-question, self-assessment paper that takes about ten minutes to complete.[4] It is useful to know what your own style is as a teacher so that if you have a trainee who has a very different style from your own, you have insight into this and can accommodate your differences. Complete the questionnaire with others and look at the match between how you generally teach that group and their preferred styles of learning, as described earlier in this section.

Stage 3: set your priorities and define your learning objectives

You may find that students or colleagues give you feedback about your competence as an educationalist that indicates your learning needs in one or more of the eight areas of competence we have described here.

Anonymised evaluation forms from a group of students or trainees, for instance, might show you that you have not held their interest or excited their wish to know more. Therefore, your objective may be to learn more about diversifying or reorganising the way you teach or train to provide a mode of teaching or providing learning experiences to match others' learning styles.

A 360° feedback exercise (*see* page 109) from colleagues with whom you work might indicate that you fail to motivate trainees when supervising their educational programmes, or put off students considering entering your specialty area. Your objective therefore may be to learn how to motivate others.

Stage 4: make an action plan with a timetable

A simple Gantt chart like that in Figure 10.1 helps you to track what you are going to do and when.

Stage 5: evaluate your progress and disseminate the results

You might choose to evaluate and determine the outcomes of your efforts by repeating the learning needs assessment(s) with which you started. You

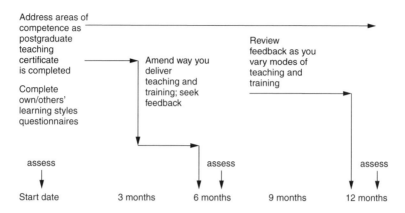

Figure 10.1:A Gantt chart for your action plan – teaching and training.

could incorporate your assessment of what has been gained into a study of another area that overlaps – perhaps as detailed in Chapter 9 on working with colleagues or one of the other chapters.

References

1Chambers R and Wall D (2000) *Teaching Made Easy.* Radcliffe Medical Press, Oxford.

2General Medical Council (2001) *Good Medical Practice.* General Medical Council, London.

3Roach S (1992) *The Human Act of Caring: a Blueprint for Health Professions.* Canadian Hospital Association Press, Ottawa.

4Honey P and Mumford A (1986) *Using Your Learning Styles.* Peter Honey, Maidenhead.

5Benner P (1984) *From Novice to Expert.* Addison-Wesley, California.

6Chambers R and See S (2002) *Accredited Professional Development Programme; facilitator's handbook.* Royal College of General Practitioners, London.

EXAMPLE DIARY SHEET FOR THIS SECTION

Diary sheet for section on teaching and training	
Stage 1: criteria and outcomes selected	To show that this doctor: 1 develops the skills, attitudes and practices of a competent teacher.
Stage 2: methods of assessment	1 Seeks feedback from students and colleagues about competence as teacher or trainer. 2 Completes learning styles questionnaire; compares own learning style and usual mode of teaching with learning styles of those being taught or trained.
Stage 3: which objectives have been selected for action this year and why	1 Feedback from students and colleagues shows that mode of teaching is generally boring. 2 Feedback also shows that doctor demotivates students and juniors about their specialty area unintentionally. The objectives are to: • learn about varying modes of delivery of teaching and training to match the needs and preferences of students and colleagues, according to their learning styles • learn how to motivate students and colleagues.
Stage 4: the action plan	Baseline feedback from students and colleagues and compare with eight areas of competence (*see* pages 120–123). Determine own and students'/colleagues' learning styles. By 3 months: register for a postgraduate teaching certificate. Learn about learning styles, teaching methods, motivation. By 6 months: experiment with various modes of delivery of teaching and training. At 12 months: review systematic feedback from teaching and training activities.
Stage 5: evaluation of progress	Discuss review of how feedback has changed through the last 12 months with a peer, e.g. at annual appraisal, or with another educationalist who might be acting as a mentor or co-mentor.

11

Probity

Introduction

This may not be a section upon which you spend much time compared to other areas of your work. You will be asked to declare in your appraisal paperwork whether you have any concerns or problems relating to probity. You should collect evidence of your probity or problem areas to back up any issues you describe.

How will you demonstrate satisfactory standards?

Remind yourself of the stages of the learning cycle for appraisal (*see* Figure A).

Stage 1: setting standards and outcomes

Look at the following criteria for a good doctor in respect of probity as listed in Box 11.1. They are derived from *Good Medical Practice* – the standards set by the General Medical Council.[1] You may want to add some others as well or expand the details given in the box.

Box 11.1: Criteria for probity

You should:

1 ensure that information about services you provide is factual and verifiable, and conforms with the law and with guidance issued by the Advertising Standards Agency
2 be able to justify any information that you publish about the quality of your services

continued overleaf

---

3   publish information about your services in such a way that it does not exploit patients' vulnerability or lack of medical knowledge or put pressure on people to use a service

4   be honest and trustworthy when writing references, reports, completing or signing forms, or providing evidence in litigation or other formal inquiries; this includes not providing documents which are misleading because they omit relevant information

5   be honest and open in any financial arrangements with patients, including agreeing fees and charges for treatment or services for you or another doctor

6   not encourage patients to give, lend or bequeath money or gifts to you

7   act in your patients' best interests when making referrals and providing or arranging treatment or care; declare any financial interests in hospitals, nursing homes and other medical organisations and do not pressure patients to accept private treatment

8   be honest in financial and commercial dealings with employers, insurers and other organisations or individuals

9   avoid treating patients in an institution in which you or members of your immediate family have financial or commercial interests. If you do so, declare any conflicts of interest and, if a specialist, do not accept patients unless they are referred by another doctor who continues to take overall responsibility for managing the patient's care.

Stage 2: identify your learning needs

You may decide to incorporate your learning needs assessment in respect of probity together with one of the other areas, so that you cover more than one in a single assessment. For this type of combined assessment, you might use:

* examination of patient records (*see* Chapter 13) to determine if patient care meets recommended standards of probity
* significant event audit (*see* Chapter 9).

Learning needs assessment techniques that are particularly suitable for use in determining standards in relation to probity are:

* evaluation of consent issues to look at how you deal with, or pass on, information to others
* a review of how reports, forms and enquiries are completed.

These two methods are considered in more detail below.

(i) Evaluation of consent issues to look at how you deal with, or pass on, information to others

People should feel free to decline to consent to participate in treatment or private healthcare (or whatever is the matter under debate) without feeling that this will prejudice the quality of the care or attention they receive from you in future.[2] Consent is only meaningful if someone receives a full explanation of the intervention or alternatives proposed. In the case of a survey, for instance, you should explain why you are carrying out the initiative and whether participating in the initial exercise to which you are inviting them could lead to you wanting them to co-operate with more in-depth work.

The right to grant or withhold consent presupposes the mental capacity or ability to do so. There is an association between competency or capacity to be well informed and the degree of previous education. You should be aware of this and act accordingly by recognising the inability of some individuals to provide informed consent – those who have educational, social and cultural reasons that limit their understanding of complex issues.

Assessing your learning needs might include the meaning and practice of obtaining informed consent, or carrying out an evaluation of the extent to which patients whose consent you have obtained felt that you had informed them of the various options. The issues of consent that you could look at in respect of probity would be financial and commercial dealing, or those in relation to research (*see* Chapter 13). You might ask relevant patients for feedback using a semi-structured interview schedule that you and an independent colleague have previously agreed. Ten such patients should give you a fair idea.

(ii) A review of how reports, forms and enquiries are completed

Organise such a review as a significant event audit (*see* Chapter 9). Choose the nature of the reports, forms or enquiries that you think will yield most information – your activity might be in relation to a problem or concern that has cropped up and you want to check that there are no similar problems. For instance, an ex-employee may have complained that the reference you gave did not do justice to his or her strengths and talents. Or an employer might have complained that the reference you gave for an ex-member of staff that painted him or her in glowing terms had omitted information about lack of punctuality or frequent sickness absence.

In the case of supplying references, your standards will be taken from the criteria in Box 11.1. You might compare the last five references that you have supplied against these criteria. One method might be to rewrite all five without looking at the originals, trying to be as informative and fair as possible. You might find upon comparison with the originals that there were omissions which you regret with hindsight. You may have blind spots (*see* the text on the JoHari Window, page 70) and it may be difficult to gain another's view of how you have constructed the references – unless you ask the people about whom the references were written to critique them, or the new employers to whom you sent the references to comment after a time interval. It may be easier to ask others to comment on your standards of completeness or the accuracy of reports or enquiries that are not about such personal information as are individuals' references.

Stage 3: set your priorities and define your learning objectives

Group together and summarise your learning needs from the exercises you have carried out. Grade them according to the priority you set. You may put one at a higher priority because it fits in with learning needs established from another section, or put another lower because it does not fit in with other activities that you will put into your learning plan for the next 12 months. If you have identified a learning need by several different methods of assessment then it will have a higher priority than something only identified once.

It may be that you have not uncovered any problems or issues with probity and feel that you can make a statement to that effect – so that you do not have any learning objectives.

You could have found that you are not sure how to write an impartial and comprehensive reference when you have concerns about an individual's performance. Or it may be that your learning needs assessments have shown that your patients have not understood your explanations when you have described options before requesting they sign their consent.

Stage 4: make an action plan with a timetable

Decide on what method of learning is most appropriate to your task.

A simple Gantt chart like the one in Figure 11.1 helps you to track what you are going to do and when.

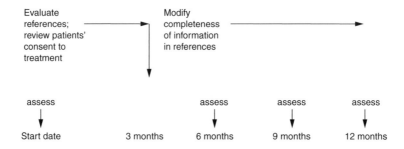

Figure 11.1: A Gantt chart for your action plan – probity.

Stage 5: evaluate your progress

You might choose to evaluate and determine the outcomes of your efforts by repeating the assessment that you started with. You might value the feedback from colleagues about your improved skills or performance in writing references or obtaining consent. A second review or evaluation may confirm your progress.

EXAMPLE DIARY SHEET FOR THIS SECTION

Diary sheet for section on probity EXAMPLE 1	
Stage 1: criteria and outcomes selected	To show that this doctor: 1 provides accurate and complete references 2 obtains well-informed patients' consent in relation to any financial or commercial matters.
Stage 2: methods of assessment	1 Evaluation of five example references; following significant event audit after complaint of unfair reference by previous employee. 2 Peer review of how well informed were patients who gave consent.
Stage 3: which needs have been selected for action this year and objectives of the action plan	1 References excluded some relevant information about problems with performance in two cases. 2 No breaches found in fully informing patients before they signed consent. The objective is to: • learn to provide full, fair and factual references.
Stage 4: the action plan	Baseline assessment as above. By 6 months: have received tutorial from personnel and modified approach to supplying references so that they are complete and factual rather than biased and subjective. At 12 months: evaluation of last two references carried out as for Stage 2.
Stage 5: evaluation of progress and dissemination	Run a tutorial for others about good practice in providing references.

References

1   General Medical Council (2001) *Good Medical Practice*. General Medical Council, London.

2   Chambers R (2000) *Involving Patients and the Public*. Radcliffe Medical Press, Oxford.

12

Management activity

Introduction

All doctors have responsibilities to use resources wisely. Some doctors will lead teams, others are part of them. The principal concern for all doctors, even when working in a management role, is the care, treatment and safety of patients. They also have a duty to their colleagues, the organisation in which they work and the wider community. Conflicts may arise when the needs of individual patients and those of the wider community cannot all be met in full. These difficulties have no easy solution.

Box 12.1:

Dr Balance had to decide how to use the staff to best advantage in the community clinics. There were not enough people to staff all the clinics at the present frequency, and no more could be employed. She could reduce the weekly clinics to every fortnight – but that would be confusing for the users and only reduce costs a little. She could shut some of the clinics that had few users – but that would disadvantage those who lived some distance from other clinics. She arranged for information on the postcodes of the clinic users to be collated and for a questionnaire to determine the views of users and staff. She consulted with staff and other managers and used a bus map to decide which clinics were best situated to serve the maximum number of users. Despite all the consultations, there were many complaints from staff and users when two of the least used and most inaccessible clinics were closed.

Clinical governance requires teamworking at all levels of the organisation with multi-professional consultation, education and training. Managers need to give effective leadership as well as enable the correct mix of team members. Managers create the culture for change and usually control the resources through which change can occur.

Managing people does not come naturally and needs to be worked at like any other skill. The best way to discover what motivates people is to ask them. Some will want more money, others more time, some more flexibility in their work schedule, others more challenging jobs. Observe how each person responds to the rewards you can offer. Remember that concerns expressed by one person about the performance of another person or organisation are not always well founded – investigate first to establish the facts, but do this without delay.

Start with the positive and with the small things. Most of us are not making earthshattering advances every day. Incentives that work include:

- personal or written congratulations from a respected colleague or immediate superior
- public recognition, e.g. announcement of success at team meetings
- recognising that the last job was well done and asking for an opinion of the next one
- providing specific and frequent feedback (positive first)
- providing information on how the task has affected the performance of the organisation or management of a patient
- encouragement to increase knowledge and skills to do even better
- making time to listen to ideas, complaints or difficulties
- learning from mistakes and making visible changes.

Doctors who take part in corporate decisions are not accountable to the General Medical Council for those decisions, only for their own conduct. However, they must take action if they believe patients are at risk of serious harm because of those decisions, other management actions or the actions of colleagues. You can obtain advice on such action from experienced colleagues, your defence organisation, professional bodies and from the General Medical Council. Occasionally, when all other avenues have been exhausted, you may need to consider making your concerns publicly known, having taken advice from your defence organisation if confidentiality is likely to be compromised in any way.

Doctors who work in public health have to base their advice on the best interests of the population and make the health of that population their first concern. They have to balance this with responsibility to their employers and the best ways to effect change. Occupational health professionals have to take into account their responsibilities to their employers, to groups of employees and to individuals. Sometimes these responsibilities will conflict and you can obtain advice from the relevant professional organisations.

However small or large your management responsibilities are, make sure that you can carry them out competently.

How will you demonstrate satisfactory standards?

Remind yourself of the stages of the learning cycle for appraisal (*see* Figure A).

Stage 1: setting standards and outcomes

Look at the following criteria for management activity listed in Box 12.2. They are derived from *Management in Health Care: the role of doctors* – standards set by the General Medical Council.[1] You may want to add some others as well or expand the details given in the box.

Box 12.2: Criteria for management activity

You should:

1 contribute to providing a work environment that allows everyone to fulfil their professional duties
2 ensure that care is provided and supervised by staff who have appropriate levels of competence
3 ensure that working methods and the work environment conform to health and safety legislation and that safe working practices are followed
4 provide, or co-operate with, complaints procedures that are prompt, fair and thorough
5 ensure that medical colleagues are aware of the standards of practice required by the General Medical Council and professional bodies
6 ensure that colleagues in other disciplines are aware of the professional guidance issued by their professional and regulatory bodies
7 help to provide a learning culture so that best use is made of opportunities for education and training
8 disseminate clinical effectiveness information
9 arrange for appropriate supervision of staff and colleagues
10 promote communication within teams, be clear about the roles and responsibilities of each team member, give support and aid development as required
11 monitor and review to improve the quality of the care provided in the work environment
12 be able to explain and justify your decisions.

Stage 2: identify your learning needs

You may decide to incorporate your learning needs assessment for management activity together with one of the other areas, so that you cover more than one in a single assessment. For this type of combined assessment, you might use:

- self-assessment (*see* Chapter 6) using a rating scale to assess your skills and attitudes
- reflective practice identifying your learning needs, team or patients' needs (*see* Chapter 6)
- patient feedback or patient satisfaction surveys (*see* Chapter 8)
- significant event audit, constructive feedback with peer observation, 360° feedback, role description, identifying team difficulties (*see* Chapter 9)
- examination of patient records (*see* Chapter 13) to determine if patient care meets recommended standards.

Learning needs assessment techniques that are particularly suitable for use in determining standards in management activity are:

- audit of protocols and guidelines
- review of delegation
- monitoring of availability and access to care, of safety and maintenance of equipment and of the environment, etc.
- patient complaint reviews to identify the problems that have led to a complaint being made.

These four methods are described in detail below.

(i) Audit of protocols and guidelines

Audit is 'the method used by health professionals to assess, evaluate, and improve the care of patients in a systematic way, to enhance their health and quality of life'.[2] The five steps of the audit cycle are to:

1 describe the criteria and standards you are trying to achieve
2 measure your current performance of how well you are providing care or services in an objective way
3 compare your performance against the criteria and standards
4 identify the need for change – to performance, adjustment of criteria or standards, resources, available data
5 make any required changes as necessary and re-audit later.

Performance is often broken down into the three aspects of structure, process and outcome for the purposes of audit; this approach was recommended by Donabedian.[3]

Structural audits might concern resources such as equipment, premises, skills, people etc. Process audits focus on what was done to the patient, for instance, clinical protocols and guidelines. Audits of outcomes consider the impact of care or services on the patient and might include patient satisfaction, health gains, and effectiveness of care or services.

The direction of clinical audit should be to promote:

- a clear patient focus
- greater multi-professional working
- an intersectoral approach across primary, secondary and continuing care boundaries
- close links with educational and professional development
- the integration of information about clinical effectiveness, cost effectiveness, variations in practice, outcome measurement and critical appraisal skills.[4]

You might determine your learning needs (and those of other team members) by collecting examples of all the protocols or guidelines that exist somewhere in the workplace together and rationalising them so that you have a common set. There are bound to be associated learning needs with taking this common approach to enable everyone to be aware of them, understand their roles and responsibilities for the various pathways in your everyday work, and be able to adhere to the protocols or guidelines, or justify any deviation.

You could also use audit to examine your standards for any other activities. Audit becomes an easy procedure, particularly when information is stored on a computer in a way that is well coded, accurate and retrievable. Once the parameters for a computerised audit are set up, it is easy to repeat the audit cycle to determine the impact of the changes you make. Be critical of the results, however. Just because you can count something, it does not mean that the results are significant in their own right. The results must be considered in the context from which they were obtained, especially if the results do not agree with common sense – so look at how the data were obtained. You may find significant errors and omissions from which you can also learn.

(ii) Review of delegation

This is often one of the most difficult tasks to do well. Work through the checklist in Box 12.3 to establish whether you have any learning needs in this area.

Box 12.3: Delegation skills checklist

1 I'm too busy to find the time to show   Usually Sometimes Occasionally
someone else how to do it.

2 I don't trust anyone else to do it as   Usually Sometimes Occasionally
well as I can.

3 I don't know what the capabilities   Usually Sometimes Occasionally
of other people are but I have to
give the tasks to them anyway.

continued overleaf

4	I want to keep control over what is happening so I have to be involved all the time.	Usually Sometimes Occasionally
5	When I ask people to do things, they keep coming back to ask me questions about how much responsibility they can take, or what they should do next.	Usually Sometimes Occasionally
6	When I ask people to do things, they say that they are too busy, or they don't do the tasks quickly enough, so I end up doing them myself.	Usually Sometimes Occasionally
7	I have so many out-of-work responsibilities that I feel too stressed to do my work properly.	Usually Sometimes Occasionally

If you answered 'usually' or 'sometimes' to most of these questions, you need to learn more about skills in delegation. Your job is to concentrate on the things you can do and others cannot. Involving others in understanding what needs to be done, what responsibility they should take and the timescale for action helps them to feel part of an organisation that functions well.

(iii) Monitoring

Regular activities require action and review. Systems and procedures require regular monitoring for good patient care and the smooth running of the organisation. You might monitor the following:

- Systems for the purchase, servicing and maintenance of equipment. Make sure that the people who have responsibility for checking equipment have deputies who know their role in the case of absence or sickness.
- Staff health – e.g. that you have procedures for ensuring that immunisation against tetanus, rubella and hepatitis is checked before employment and at the recommended intervals.
- Confidentiality – to make sure that new staff are aware of the rules and that breaches of confidentiality do not occur.
- Safety and maintenance of the premises – that they are clean and present no hazards to staff or patients.
- Systems and procedures for referrals, letters and reports, notification of results of investigations, etc.
- Waiting times – to see a health professional from the time of the appointment or admission to the time a patient is seen, the next available appointment slot, the interval before investigations or treatments are performed.

(iv) Complaints

An effective complaints procedure should be in place and used properly. Records of complaints and how they are handled should be kept and examined to see if any pattern emerges. Even when a complaint is shown to have been unjustified, it often represents a failure of communication. Sometimes this is inevitable (for instance, if a patient has become paranoid or otherwise mentally unbalanced), but more often it is due to a lack of thought or consideration of the other person's knowledge or point of view.

Complaints may shine a spotlight on all sorts of deficiencies in the provision of patient care, and may also specifically illuminate problems in your style or conduct of management.

Box 12.4:

Dr Govern was told by one of the nurses that a cleaner had complained to her that she had found a sharps box tipped over with its contents spilled on the floor. The nurse said it was not her responsibility to close and change the boxes. Dr Govern looked up who was responsible and found that the nurse who normally checked the sharps containers, closed and changed them, was off sick and her deputy was on holiday. A review of the procedures showed that because responsibility had been given to just two people, everyone else felt it was nothing to do with them. Several other checks were found to suffer from the same deficiency. The objective here was to make everyone aware of their responsibility to comply with safety requirements and how they might do so.

A complaint may show that the time between the receipt of an informal complaint and your response is too long and it has escalated into a formal complaint. You need to tighten up the procedure to avoid this occurring again.

Stage 3: set your priorities and define your learning objectives

Look back at Stage 1 for your standards for management activity. Match your learning needs with one or more of the criteria in Box 12.2 or others you have set yourself.

You may have found that there were many protocols and guidelines in existence, but that most staff did not know of their existence or, if they did, were unable to access them easily. Adherence to such documents is likely to be poor under these circumstances! Therefore, even before you can audit whether protocols and guidelines are being followed, your objective will be to sort out with your colleagues and staff which ones should be in use and how they will be accessed.

Your skills at delegation may be poor. You want to do it all yourself and keep control, but in the process feel overwhelmed and unable to function properly. Your objectives may be to establish the competencies of the staff and colleagues to whom you can delegate, so that you feel able to do so.

Your monitoring exercise may have turned up deficiencies in your systems and procedures. Together with the team of people involved, new responsibilities may need to be taken, or procedures altered.

Stage 4: make an action plan with a timetable

Decide on what method of learning is most appropriate to your task.

Describe how you will carry out your learning tasks and what you will do by a specified time. Say how your learning will be applied and how and when it will be evaluated. Build in some staging posts so that you do not suddenly get to the end of 12 months and discover that you have only done half of your plan.

A simple Gantt chart like the one in Figure 12.1 helps you to track what you are going to do and when.

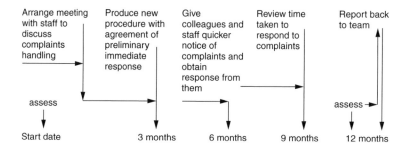

Figure 12.1:   A Gantt chart for your action plan – management activity.

Stage 5: evaluate your progress

You might choose to evaluate and determine the outcomes of your efforts by repeating the assessment with which you started. You might value the feedback from colleagues about your improved skills or attitudes. A patient satisfaction measure carried out for other purposes may confirm your progress. You might evaluate the changes by the degree to which your own level of stress or dissatisfaction has been reduced.

References

1 General Medical Council (2001) *Management in Health Care: the role of doctors.* General Medical Council, London.

2 Irvine D and Irvine S (eds) (1991) *Making Sense of Audit.* Radcliffe Medical Press, Oxford. Out of print.

3 Donabedian A (1966) Evaluating the quality of medical care. *Millbank Memorial Fund Quarterly.* **44**: 166–204.

4 NHS Executive (1996) *Clinical Audit in the NHS. Using clinical audit in the NHS: a position statement.* NHS Executive, Leeds.

EXAMPLE DIARY SHEET FOR THIS SECTION

Diary sheet for section on management activity	
Stage 1: criteria and outcomes selected	To show that this doctor: 1 provides a learning culture 2 disseminates clinical effectiveness material.
Stage 2: methods of assessment	1 Records of identification of learning needs and the opportunities and facilitation provided. 2 Feedback from staff and colleagues. 3 Audit of changes using clinical effectiveness material to identify unsatisfactory practices.
Stage 3: which needs have been selected for action this year (and why) and objectives of the action plan	1 Feedback indicates that overload of service commitments prevents access to learning in working hours; identification of opportunities for learning and facilitation regarded as poor. 2 Audit of use of clinical effectiveness material satisfactory and will be continued. The objective is to: • provide learning opportunities during working hours.
Stage 4: the action plan	Baseline assessment as above. By 3 months: discussion with library staff and health professionals about how to provide online look-up provision in working hours. By 6 months: piloting of access to TRIP and MEDLINE from all computer stations with web access; rolling programme of training staff provided by library staff in work time. At 9 months: records of use and feedback suggest rollout to other sites needed; business plan to convert non-web-connected terminals to web-enabled. At 12 months: two-thirds of computer terminals now web-enabled and use of online look-up increasing.
Stage 5: evaluation of progress and dissemination	1 Training of staff and use of online look-up monitored by library staff. 2 Monitoring of use and feedback from users suggested system worked well and needed extending. 3 Partial success by 12 months but longer time needed to assess progress and usefulness.

13

Research

Introduction

This may not be a section upon which you spend much time compared to other areas of your work if you are not actively involved in research. It may be that you are not taking part in any research activity at all – not even referring patients to others' research projects or helping with a colleague's research project in any way. If so, you need to do nothing more than declare that you do not participate in research.

You may be merely helping others with their research – in which case many of the criteria in Box 13.1 will apply to you.

Doctors with special interests or responsibilities for research, or for teaching and training others about research, may weight the time and effort they spend on their personal and professional development towards research, and collect substantial evidence for their appraisal portfolio in relation to this section. All the criteria in Box 13.1 will apply to these doctors.

Doctors who combine a part-time post as a researcher with clinical practice will produce a more substantial body of evidence about their research practice as opposed to doctors whose research activities are an incidental part of their daily jobs. The doctors may demonstrate how they have become more knowledgeable, skilled and proficient as researchers and how they are able to apply their work and disseminate their results to others.

If you are responsible for conducting research or organising a research study, you will be asked to include any relevant documents in your appraisal paperwork, such as records of any research that is ongoing or was completed in the previous year, records of funding arrangements or appropriate ethical approval.

How will you demonstrate satisfactory standards?

Remind yourself of the stages of the learning cycle for appraisal (*see* Figure A).

Stage 1: setting standards and outcomes

Look at the following criteria for research as listed in Box 13.1. They are derived from *Good Medical Practice* and *Research: the role and responsibilities of doctors* – the standards set by the General Medical Council.[1,2] You may want to add some others as well or expand the details given in the box.

Box 13.1: Criteria for research

You should:

1 put the care and safety of patients first when participating in research
2 ensure that approval has been obtained for research from an independent research ethics committee and that patients have given informed consent
3 conduct all research in an ethical manner, with honesty and integrity
4 be satisfied that the foreseeable risks will not outweigh the potential benefits to patients in therapeutic research
5 be satisfied that the potential benefits from the development of treatments and furthering of knowledge far outweigh any foreseeable risks to participants in non-therapeutic research
6 ensure that patients or volunteers understand that they are being asked to participate in research and that the results are not predictable
7 respect participants' rights to confidentiality
8 record and report results accurately
9 do your best to complete research projects involving patients or volunteers or ensure that they are completed by others (except where harms or risks are expected)
10 keep GPs and other clinicians who are responsible for the participant's care informed of the participant's involvement, with the participant's consent
11 follow the research protocol approved by the research ethics committee.[3]

Stage 2: identify your learning needs

You may decide to incorporate your learning needs assessment in respect of research together with one of the other sections, so that you cover more than one in a single assessment. For this type of combined assessment, you might use

- examination of patient records to determine if patient care meets recommended standards of probity (*see* Chapter 13)
- significant event audit (*see* Chapter 9).

Learning needs assessment techniques that are particularly suitable for use in determining standards in relation to research are:

- a review of records of participants in a research study

- a review of the adherence of the researchers to the study protocol agreed by the research ethics committee.

These two methods are considered in more detail below.

(i) A review of records of participants in a research study

This might be undertaken as an audit (*see* Chapter 7) of the records to check that all details are being entered in study forms as measurements are made or results come in. You might, for instance, audit that the written consent of patients participating in the research study is consistently recorded, or that records are being stored securely so that participants' details remain confidential.

(ii) A review of the adherence of the researchers to the study protocol agreed by the research ethics committee

As a senior researcher you would be responsible for the conduct of your research and for ensuring that any research undertaken follows the agreed study protocol.

You might undertake a review at intervals to check that you and other associated researchers are following best practice and the protocol in such issues as:

- identifying and recruiting patients and volunteers to participate in the research
- explaining the research and the associated risks and benefits, then seeking informed consent
- sampling
- carrying out the research method according to the study design
- keeping and storing records
- helping health and social care professionals to ensure that participants receive appropriate care while they are involved in research
- reporting any failures or adverse events
- handling and analysing the results
- minimising biases
- completing the research study and writing up the report(s).

Stage 3: set your priorities and define your learning objectives

Group together and summarise your learning needs from the exercises you have carried out. Grade them according to the priorities you set. You may put one at a higher priority because it fits in with learning needs established from another section, or put another lower because it does not fit in with other activities that you will put into your learning plan for the next 12 months. If you have identified a learning need by several different methods of assessment then it will have a higher priority than something identified only once.

It may be that you have not uncovered any problems or issues with research and feel that you can make a statement to that effect – so that you do not have any learning objectives.

You could have found that your record-keeping needs improvement or that you are not adhering to best practice in the undertaking of research in an intentional or unconscious way. The research governance framework being introduced for health and social care describes best practice for all those involved in research from the perspectives of all involved: participants, researchers, principal investigator, funder, sponsor, employing organisation, care organisation, responsible care professional and research ethics committee.[3]

Therefore, formulate the objectives of your personal development plan accordingly.

Stage 4: make an action plan with a timetable

Decide on what method of learning is most appropriate to your task.

A simple Gantt chart like the one in Figure 13.1 helps you to track what you are going to do and when.

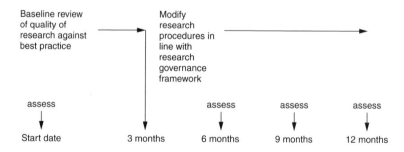

Figure 13.1:   A Gantt chart for your action plan – research.

Stage 5: evaluate your progress

You might choose to evaluate and determine the outcome of your efforts by repeating the assessment that you started with. A second review or evaluation may confirm your progress.

EXAMPLE DIARY SHEET FOR THIS SECTION

Diary sheet for section on research	
Stage 1: criteria and outcomes selected	To show that this doctor: 1 adheres to best practice in the conduct of research.
Stage 2: methods of assessment	1 Review of records of participants in research. 2 Review of how study was conducted, comparing what actually happened against agreed study protocol.
Stage 3: which needs have been selected for action this year and objectives of the action plan	1 Review of participants' records show breach of confidentiality occurred. 2 Breaches of research protocol demonstrate learning needs about meaning of research governance, e.g. scientific design sacrificed for expediency. The objectives are to: • learn about the requirements of research governance and how systems and procedures can be set up in partnership with others • continue to preserve best practice in the conduct of research.
Stage 4: the action plan	Baseline assessment as above. By 6 months: have received tutorial from lead on research governance in trust along with other responsible researchers. Agree shared systems and procedures for monitoring quality of research and adherence to agreed research study protocols. At 12 months: re-evaluation of adherence to study protocol at key stages of research.
Stage 5: evaluation of progress and dissemination	Continue to monitor quality of research and collect evidence to be able to demonstrate quality to others. Run a tutorial for others involved in research locally about good practice in conducting research in accordance with requirements of research governance.[3]

References

1   General Medical Council (2001) *Good Medical Practice*. General Medical Council, London.

2   General Medical Council (2001) *Research: the role and responsibility of doctors*. General Medical Council, London.

3   Department of Health (2001) *Research Governance Framework for Health and Social Care*. Department of Health, London.

14

Health

This may not be a section upon which you spend much time compared to other areas of your work. You will be asked to declare in your appraisal paperwork whether you have any concerns or problems relating to your health. You should collect evidence for any problem areas to back up any issues you describe.

Look at the following criterion for health listed in Box 14.1. It is derived from *Good Medical Practice*.

Box 14.1: Criterion for health

You should:

1 take and follow advice from a consultant in occupational health or other suitably qualified colleague on whether and how you should modify your practice, if you know that you have a serious condition which you could pass on to patients, or that your judgement or performance could be significantly affected by a condition or illness or its treatment.

This section does not require you to follow the five stages of the learning cycle as other sections do. If you are able to make a self-declaration that you have no health problems of this kind, then you do not need to focus on collecting evidence to demonstrate your health nor plan to learn more about this topic in your personal development plan.

If you recognise that you *are* suffering from a serious condition or illness or that treatment for a health problem is putting patient safety and well-being at risk, you should consult your general practitioner and/or an occupational health specialist as appropriate. If you continue to work, you should be able to justify your actions and decisions.

15

Make a logical plan to achieve revalidation through successful appraisals

Advantages of a logical framework

The logical framework has been used for project planning for decades as an approach to planning and monitoring overseas development programmes.[1] Recently, the logical framework has been used in the health service for planning and evaluating health action projects.[2,3]

You could regard preparing for appraisals and undertaking the associated learning and work as a project and use the logical framework (log frame) to think out your ultimate aims – such as being an effective doctor and achieving revalidation. The approach will force you to consider the assumptions you are making in setting out your action plan. You will be able to monitor your progress and pre-empt obstructions to your plans. The log frame is an aid to thinking, rather than a series of procedures to which you slavishly adhere, so we have adapted the framework to help you plan the operational aspects of your appraisal 'project' – what, when, why and how.[1]

Why has your good resolution to compose and carry out a personal development plan failed in the past? Is it because *carrying out* your resolution was more complex a matter than simply making the resolution? Other factors may have intruded that you had not foreseen. Your vision might have been unrealistic; you may not have had the skills to identify what you needed to learn, as opposed to what you fancied learning, or the time or money for the planned learning activities. You may have mistakenly presumed that your colleagues or staff would support you in applying what you learnt and found that they were reluctant to make changes that affected their work. Or you may just not have got round to it!

Why not think of using a project management approach to prepare for appraisal and carry out the plan you agree with your appraiser – and map out activities, outputs, purpose and goals. The log frame approach handles the complex nature of making and undertaking an action plan to prepare for and take the contents of the appraisal agreement forward across all the dimensions of your working life. The framework encourages you to set specific goals. It helps you to analyse your weaknesses and guides you to consider the assumptions you are making – in the details of your plan of action or in pursuing your goals. This approach helps you to realise the interactions between what you can do for yourself and external factors that either enhance or hinder your plans. The log frame helps you to set out realistic milestones and decide in advance how you will monitor your progress. It helps you to:

* organise your thinking
* relate your planned activities to the results you can expect
* set performance indicators for yourself
* allocate responsibilities for yourself and to others – within your practice, department or organisation.

The structure of the log frame consists of a 4×4 matrix. The rows represent the project objectives and the means to achieve them (vertical logic). The columns indicate how you can verify that you have achieved your objectives (horizontal logic) and the assumptions you are making.

The vertical logic

Step 1: define your overall **goal** – the reason for you undertaking the 'project'. This is the ultimate objective of your appraisal. Phrase this in your own words. An example might be 'to be an effective doctor' or 'to achieve revalidation'.

Step 2: define the **purpose** of the 'project'. The purpose is the reason why you are proposing to carry out the project – what it will achieve once it is completed within your timescale and what impact you hope to make. It is the motivation behind the outputs of the project. An example might be 'successful appraisal each year' – to do this you will have satisfactorily implemented the learning and work plans you agreed with your appraisers at each appraisal. It keeps the project more streamlined if you only have one purpose.

Step 3: define the **outputs** for achieving the purpose of the 'project'. These are what you want the project to achieve – the specific end results that will be achieved when the planned activities are carried out. An example might be 'appraisal portfolio approved by appraiser'. Achieving the outputs should be within your control.

Step 4: define the **activities** that you will undertake in order to achieve each output, and the resources available. Activities define how you will carry out your project. Examples might be 'compose a personal development plan' or 'attend training workshop on a relevant topic'. You should expect to undertake three to seven activities for every output you hope to accomplish (*see* Table 15.2 for an example).

The log frame structure is based upon the concept of cause and effect. The vertical logic is based on a sequence of causal relationships starting from the bottom upwards. There is a logical relationship between activities and outputs, outputs and the purpose, the purpose and the goal. **If** specific activities are carried out, **then** certain outputs will be produced. If the outputs you describe are produced, then the declared purpose will be achieved. If the purpose is achieved, your goal should be attained. Thus, reading from the bottom upwards:

GOAL

then ↑

if PURPOSE

then ↑

if OUTPUTS

then ↑

if ACTIVITIES

The first three levels of activities, outputs and purpose are specific to the 'project' itself – in this case, successful appraisal – whereas your goal is at a higher level – such as 'being an effective doctor'. For the purposes of this 'project' we will adopt 'achieving revalidation' as the ultimate goal.

Evaluate your results sequentially, from the bottom upwards. You cannot logically evaluate the *outputs* of your activities without first monitoring that the *activities* have been carried out and achieved as planned. Similarly, you cannot expect to obtain the improvements described in your *purpose* without the *outputs* having been achieved first.

The horizontal logic

Horizontal logic underlies the way you measure the effectiveness of your plan. Specify how you will measure progress for each of the four levels of the vertical logic: the activities, outputs, purpose and goal. Use concrete terms, rather than vague measures, as tangible indicators of progress. These indicators should have the following qualities:

- clearly describe how the achievement of the activity, output or purpose contributes to the success of the project
- focus on what is important for the purpose or overall goal
- clearly relate to the activity, output, purpose or goal with which they are associated

- be of sufficient number and in enough detail to measure activities, outputs, purpose and goal adequately
- be specific to an activity, output, purpose or goal
- be objectively verifiable so that two independent observers measure achievement in the same way – quantitative or qualitative in nature.

The indicator might be direct (e.g. audit results from monitoring that learning has been undertaken and applied) or indirect (e.g. number and type of training courses you attended).

Don't forget, as before, these indicators should be SMART (specific, measurable, achievable, realistic and time-limited).

Next, decide how you will verify that all the specified indicators have been achieved. You might gather simple data as part of your project, or refer to sources of information such as reports, surveys, official documents, notes of meetings or a review of case studies over time.

Box 15.1:

'For each level of the vertical logic there will be a set of objectively verifiable indicators which are appropriate to the objectives at that level and which constitute proof of achievement at that level.'[1]

Important assumptions

You know that it is very unlikely that your plans will go forward without a hitch, but that doesn't stop you assuming that you will progress smoothly. In reality, things crop up unexpectedly which obstruct or delay your progress.

The assumptions that you describe in your log frame include factors or conditions that could affect your progress with the project or its overall success, over which you have no, or limited, control. For the overseas development projects for which the log frame has been used, these might include external factors such as unexpected bad weather or an earthquake.

For you, planning for an appraisal, examples of major external factors beyond your control are new government requirements about reorganising your specialty or the passing of new legislation for what has to be demonstrated at appraisal or to achieve revalidation. More minor assumptions might be the extent of co-operation that is forthcoming from other members of your team or the managers in your department, practice or trust. These will affect whether you are able to undertake the activities you plan, or achieve the outputs or purpose in your log frame.

As well as the unexpected factors that might spoil your plans, you may be assuming too much. It may be that, for instance, you have insufficient knowledge and skills to carry out the activities you envisage, or you might not have forecast the extent of resources needed to implement your ideas.

There may be other risks to your planned timetable too. You may not have thought through the consequences of your plans – the opportunity costs if you switch the way that resources are allocated (time, effort, money etc.) in line with your action plan. You may not have predicted the new stress-provoking factors that might arise from the revised systems and procedures you establish in the course of carrying out your plan; they may interfere with your ability to apply what you learn or perform at work.

Getting started

Read through the steps below and work through the thinking behind how we have put the log frame together. Before you start, note down all the people who will have some influence on the progress or viability of your plan for appraisal, throughout the lifetime of your 'project'. They might be:

- other team members
- managers in your department, practice or trust
- staff to whom you delegate work
- your GP tutor or clinical or college tutor
- people who delegate work to you
- people for whom you are responsible
- your appraiser.

You will need to anticipate how they will influence your plan – enhancing or limiting progress. Consider how they will interact with you and include them in the activities of your log frame, or in the assumptions that you make. You will be taking account of their influence, by harnessing their help or preventing them from obstructing you, in the nature of the activities that you include in your plan.

The worked example that we develop below illustrates the processes that you need to adopt to make up a log frame. The contents of the example log frame are an illustration of the thinking behind a log frame and are not prescriptive. You should use the evolving framework as a guide rather than lift the example 'off the peg' for your own requirements. Much of the learning and benefits from a log frame arise from the preparatory work in putting it together and thinking through the factors that are individual to you and that will enhance or prevent your progress. They will be peculiar to you, your network of people and your circumstances.

We have not included every detail about possible assumptions or potential risks that might occur during such a project plan or even the numerous activities that you could undertake. To do so would have resulted in such an extent of background detail that it would be difficult for the reader to distinguish 'must do' information from 'could do' detail. You will be able to include more minor information about risks and assumptions yourself – the columns of a completed log frame that is undertaken over a year or more often stretch to over three or four sides of A4 paper.[3]

Have a first go at establishing the vertical logic

Step 1: have a go at writing down the goal of your 'project'. In Table 15.1, this is 'To achieve successful revalidation'. You might want to take a wider view and consider that your ultimate goal is to 'be an effective doctor' or 'provide better healthcare for patients and the community'.

Step 2: have a go at writing down the purpose of your 'project'. In Table 15.1, this is 'Successful appraisal each year'.

Step 3: have a go at writing down the outputs of your 'project' that taken together will achieve your purpose. These are really intermediate achievements in your progress plan. In Table 15.1 these are: 'action from previous personal development plan (PDP) successfully concluded', 'appraisal portfolio approved by appraiser and primary care organisation (PCO) or hospital management' and 'successful appraisal interview'. Now you need to challenge yourself: are there gaps; are these three outputs appropriate for your purpose?

Step 4: have a go at writing down the activities that you think should achieve each output. In Table 15.1 these are given as: 'identify learning needs', 'compose PDP', 'undertake learning of PDP', 'understand meaning of the seven headings in the General Medical Council's *Good Medical Practice*' and 'seek patient feedback about own work'.

Now you should apply the 'if ... then' logic described before to test cause and effect. **If** these activities are carried out, **then** you will achieve these outputs. **If** you identify your learning needs and compose a personal development plan, **then** your appraisal portfolio will be approved ... you can see that the case is crumbling – there are missing links.

You will have to do more than simply compose a personal development plan – you will have to find ways to apply your learning and associated changes to your work practices and it will have to link in with all aspects of your roles and responsibilities in your health service work, including clinical governance, for instance. You have been assuming that composing a PDP is all that you need to do, whereas in actual fact you should have undertaken linked activities such as prioritised learning about relevant skills, located an

Table 15.1: Step 1 of building up the log frame to achieve successful appraisals and ultimately revalidation – your first attempt at planning your vertical logical pathway

	Summary	Indicators	Verification	Assumptions
Goal	To achieve successful revalidation			
Purpose	Successful appraisal each year			
Outputs (intermediate achievements)	• Action from previous PDP successfully concluded • Appraisal portfolio approved by appraiser and PCO or hospital management • Successful appraisal interview			
Activities	• Identify learning needs • Compose PDP • Undertake learning of PDP • Understand meaning of the seven headings in *Good Medical Practice* • Seek patient feedback about own work			

appropriate training course, created time to go, justified the course fees, practised the skills learnt etc.

Look again at these activities and outputs. **If** you identify your learning needs, compose a PDP and undertake learning as planned, **then** ... what? The outputs described in Table 15.1 were about your appraisal portfolio being completed and approved. There are *no* intermediary steps in the list of activities for utilising the information gathered from the patient feedback or building on your understanding of the seven headings in *Good Medical Practice* – so you need to add some more activities, as we do in Table 15.2.

Table 15.2: Step 2 of building up the log frame to achieve successful appraisals and ultimately revalidation – linking activities with outputs

	Summary	Indicators	Verification	Assumptions
Goal	To achieve successful revalidation			
Purpose	Successful appraisal each year			
Outputs (intermediate achievements)	1 Action from previous PDP successfully concluded 2 Appraisal portfolio approved by appraiser and PCO or hospital management 3 Successful appraisal interview			

continued overleaf

Table 15.2: *continued*

	Summary	*Indicators*	*Verification*	*Assumptions*
Activities	1.1 Identify learning needs			
	1.2 Seek patient feedback about own work			
	1.3 Understand meaning of the seven headings in *Good Medical Practice*			
	1.4 Prioritise learning needs and compose PDP			
	1.5 Arrange learning activities; find resources to provide cover and course fees; locate training courses			
	1.6 Practise and apply new skills			
	1.7 Monitor that learning has taken place and been applied			
	2.1 Become familiar with clinical governance plan and NHS priorities			
	2.2 Link own work to clinical governance plan			
	2.3 Make changes to systems and procedures reflecting action from PDP and links to clinical governance			
	2.4 Become familiar with requirements for organisation of appraisal paperwork and portfolio			
	2.5 Keep records of own practice as part of overall team's performance			
	2.6 Compile appraisal portfolio, updating it regularly over the year			
	2.7 Submit appraisal portfolio and paperwork to appraiser in good time			
	3.1 Arrange time and location for appraisal with appraiser			
	3.2 Arrange cover for your work for time of appraisal			
	3.3 Ensure no interruptions while appraisal takes place			
	3.4 Prepare well for appraisal – reflect on current gaps and likely future plans to discuss at appraisal			

Numbering the outputs and the activities linked to them will help you to see how **if** you undertake certain activities, **then** you will achieve specific outputs – as in Table 15.2. Making these linkages has made it more obvious that other activities have to be undertaken to achieve the outputs. Some of these have been added, in **bold**, in Table 15.2.

Now that you are starting to get the vertical logic in place, you should start thinking about what assumptions you have been making, and if there are any potential risks associated with your logical plan. Once you have recognised these, you may have to add other activities, to minimise the effects of previously unforeseen external factors. This is the stage when you should be anticipating problems that could interrupt the progress of your project action plan. You may have a blind spot about these possible problem areas, so you could usefully discuss the preliminary thinking of your project plan with someone else who might point out weaknesses you have not yet recognised, or give you information about possible external influences of which you were unaware.

Look at Table 15.3 to see some examples of assumptions that you might be making, given in **bold**. You can see that as you think through how you are going to undertake those activities and turn them into outputs, some gaps are appearing – you may be assuming, for instance, you already possess the knowledge and skills to compose a personal development plan, or that there is a clinical governance plan in place at work.

Table 15.3: Step 3 of building up the log frame to achieve successful appraisals and ultimately revalidation – adding in assumptions about your planned activities

	Summary	*Indicators*	*Verification*	*Assumptions*
Goal	To achieve successful revalidation			
Purpose	Successful appraisal each year			
Outputs (intermediate achievements)	1 Action from previous PDP successfully concluded 2 Appraisal portfolio approved by appraiser and PCO or hospital management 3 Successful appraisal interview			
Activities				**Assumes that:**
	1.1 Identify learning needs			**1.1 Know how and have skills to undertake learning needs assessment**

continued overleaf

Table 15.3: *continued*

Summary	Indicators	Verification	Assumptions
1.2 Seek patient feedback about own work			**1.2 Know how and have skills to seek patient feedback**
1.3 Understand meaning of seven headings in *GMP*			**1.3 Headings in *GMP* are unambiguous and interpreted in same way by all**
1.4 Prioritise learning needs and compose PDP			**1.4 Know how to prioritise needs and draw up PDP**
1.5 Arrange learning activities; find resources for cover/fees; locate courses			**1.5 Appropriate and affordable education and training available, matching learning needs, learning style, time**
1.6 Practise and apply new skills			**1.6 Have gained sufficient skills from courses attended and other learning to be good enough to practise**
1.7 Monitor that learning has taken place/been applied			**1.7 Know how and have skills to assess own role in delivery and quality of care and services**
2.1 Be familiar with clinical governance plan and NHS priorities			**2.1 Understand components of clinical governance**
2.2 Link own work to clinical governance plan			**2.2 Own work is congruent with clinical governance plan and can link in**
2.3 Make changes to systems and procedures from PDP and clinical governance plan			**2.3 Sufficient resources available to enable changes to be made in response to PDP and clinical governance**
2.4 Be familiar with requirements for appraisal paperwork and portfolio			**2.4 Stay up to date with any revisions to requirements**
2.5 Keep records of practice/team's performance			**2.5 Make time and capacity for record-keeping; able to distinguish individual's from team's performance**

continued opposite

Table 15.3: *continued*

Summary	Indicators	Verification	Assumptions
2.6 Compile appraisal portfolio and regularly update it			**2.6 Can make time to keep portfolio up to date and keep up resolve; others supply essential information about your practice or performance**
2.7 Submit appraisal portfolio and paperwork to appraiser			**2.7 Know who the appraiser is in good time; format of appraisal paperwork is agreed**
3.1 Arrange time/ location for appraisal with appraiser			**3.1 Can book mutually agreed time and site for appraisal; other diary commitments do not mean postponements**
3.2 Arrange cover for appraisal			**3.2 Able to cancel booked surgery or outpatient clinic or find locum cover**
3.3 Ensure no interruptions while appraisal takes place			**3.3 Appraiser and appraisee both able to arrange for emergencies to be covered by others; able to find quiet room for appraisal**
3.4 Prepare well for appraisal – reflect on gaps and plans			**3.4 PCO and hospital trust supply information about own practice and performance in good time; have opportunity to reflect on own performance; able to recognise gaps**

Examples of the types of risk that may arise are: you will waste your time attending a course or starting a distance-learning course that does not fit your needs; you identify topics you urgently need to learn more about and cannot find the right course, pitched at an appropriate level for you, that is held at a convenient time and is affordable. Other areas of risk could include: staff numbers remaining stable; significant new government directives etc.

that mean that you cannot pursue your planned priorities; a crisis at your workplace such as a flood or fire.

Therefore, the next step is to add yet more activities to anticipate the risks that you realise could happen, to reduce the likelihood of them occurring and obstructing your progress with your plan. The risks and activities given in **bold** in Table 15.4 are illustrative of a variety of risks that might occur and activities you might adopt to minimise the effects of these risks on your progress to achieving successful appraisals and ultimately revalidation. We have indicated that evolving a mutually supportive culture between colleagues (classified as activity 4 below) is a separate aspect of your logical framework, for which you would need to devise another set of activities and assumptions.

Table 15.4: Step 4 of building up the log frame to achieve successful appraisals and ultimately revalidation – add more activities to anticipate the 'risks' arising from previously planned activities and assumptions

	Summary	*Indicators*	*Verification*	*Assumptions and Risks*
Goal	To achieve successful revalidation			
Purpose	Successful appraisal each year			
Outputs (intermediate achievements)	1 Action from previous PDP successfully concluded 2 Appraisal portfolio approved by appraiser and PCO or hospital management 3 Successful appraisal interview			
Activities				Assumes that:
	1.1 Identify learning needs			1.1 Know how and have skills to undertake learning needs assessment
	1.2 Seek patient feedback about own work			1.2 Know how and have skills to seek patient feedback
	1.3 Understand meaning of seven headings in *GMP*			1.3 Headings in *GMP* are unambiguous and interpreted in same way by all
	1.4 Prioritise learning needs and compose PDP			1.4 Know how to prioritise needs and draw up PDP

continued opposite

Table 15.4: *continued*

Summary	Indicators	Verification	Assumptions and Risks
1.5 Arrange learning activities; find resources for cover/fees; locate courses			1.5 Appropriate and affordable education and training available, matching learning needs, learning style, time
1.6 Practise and apply new skills			1.6 Have gained sufficient skills from courses attended and other learning to be good enough to practise
1.7 Monitor that learning has taken place/been applied			1.7 Know how and have skills to assess own role in delivery and quality of care and services
1.8 Get course curriculum and talk to someone who has been to proposed training course			**Risk might be: 1.8 Selected course is inappropriate for you**
2.1 Be familiar with clinical governance plan and NHS priorities			2.1 Understand components of clinical governance
2.2 Link own work to clinical governance plan			2.2 Own work is congruent with clinical governance plan and can link in
2.3 Make changes to systems and procedures from PDP and clinical governance plan			2.3 Sufficient resources available to enable changes to be made in response to PDP and clinical governance
2.4 Be familiar with requirements for appraisal paperwork and portfolio			2.4 Stay up to date with any revisions to requirements
2.5 Keep records of practice/team's performance			2.5 Make time and capacity for record-keeping; able to distinguish individual's from team's performance
2.6 Compile appraisal portfolio and regularly update it			2.6 Can make time to keep portfolio up to date and keep up resolve; others supply essential information about your practice or performance

continued overleaf

Table 15.4: *continued*

	Summary	Indicators	Verification	Assumptions and Risks
	2.7 Submit appraisal portfolio and paperwork to appraiser			2.7 Know who the appraiser is in good time; format of appraisal paperwork is agreed
	2.8 Convene a meeting of managers and practitioners where priorities for clinical governance are thrashed out and consensus reached			**Risk might be: 2.8 PCO/hospital management have different priorities to you and other practitioners for clinical governance plan**
	3.1 Arrange time/ location for appraisal with appraiser			3.1 Can book mutually agreed time and site for appraisal; other diary commitments do not mean postponements
	3.2 Arrange cover for appraisal			3.2 Able to cancel the booked surgery or outpatient clinic or find locum cover
	3.3 Ensure no interruptions while appraisal takes place			3.3 Appraiser and appraisee both able to arrange for emergencies to be covered by others; able to find quiet room for appraisal
	3.4 Prepare well for appraisal – reflect on gaps and plans			3.4 PCO and hospital trust supply information about own practice and perform- ance in good time; have opportunity to reflect on own performance; able to recognise gaps
	3.5 Arrange alternative cross-cover from colleague to cover emergency if let down by current arrangements			**Risks might be: 3.5 Locum who arranged to cover your work is ill and cannot work**
	4.1 Evolve a culture of mutual support between colleagues through shared activities so that cross-cover is more likely in the event of a crisis; or your manager will try his or her hardest to find another locum (trying to evolve a supportive culture will only be possible with another set of activities/assumptions)			

The next step is to move on to specify the assumptions that you are making about attaining your outputs. Examples of these have been added in **bold** to Table 15.5.

You may, for instance, assume that you can apply what you have learnt and complete your personal development plan. However, there may be impediments to your progress, arising from aspects of the organisation or team members, of which you were previously unaware when you constructed your PDP. Therefore, consider adding another 'activity' such as an initial review of your PDP by a peer or colleagues in your team. There will be a potential risk, too, that in applying what you have learnt and making changes, you create new learning needs for others as a result of you delegating work to one of the others in the team who does not have the time or training for the additional work. The team review of your PDP which you have just added as an activity might be an opportunity to discuss ways that the team as a whole, rather than just you, can learn more about the topic you have prioritised in your PDP.

Table 15.5: Step 5 of building up the log frame to achieve successful appraisals and ultimately revalidation – adding assumptions you are making about expected outputs and adding more activities to diminish the likelihood of potential risks occurring

	Summary	*Indicators*	*Verification*	*Assumptions and Risks*
Goal	To achieve successful revalidation			
Purpose	Successful appraisal each year			
Outputs (intermediate achievements)	1 Action from previous PDP successfully concluded			**Assumes that:** **1.1 You identified key areas about which you needed to learn more** **1.2 You have applied your new knowledge and skills consistently** **1.3 You recognise how your applying learning and changing the way you practise impinges on other team members** **Risk might be:** **1.4 You have blind spots about the contents of your PDP or the way you have applied your learning**

continued overleaf

Table 15.5: *continued*

	Summary	Indicators	Verification	Assumptions and Risks
	2 Appraisal portfolio approved by appraiser and PCO or hospital management			**2.1 Your appraiser is competent to recognise good practice within appraisal portfolio and PDP** **2.2 Decision by which appraiser rates your appraisal portfolio is fair and transparent** **Risk might be that:** **2.3 Colleagues and/or staff are not agreeable to changes in their responsibilities or for their job descriptions to be revised**
	3 Successful appraisal interview			**3.1 Your appraiser is competent to run the appraisal in a constructive way** **Risk might be that:** **3.2 The appraisee and appraiser disagree about the way that plans agreed at previous appraisal have been carried out, or about extent to which limited resources have impeded progress or future priorities**
Activities				Assumes that:
	1.1 Identify learning needs			1.1 Know how and have skills to undertake learning needs assessment
	1.2 Seek patient feedback about own work			1.2 Know how and have skills to seek patient feedback
	1.3 Understand meaning of seven headings in *GMP*			1.3 Headings in *GMP* are unambiguous and interpreted in same way by all
	1.4 Prioritise learning needs and compose PDP			1.4 Know how to prioritise needs and draw up PDP

continued opposite

Table 15.5:　*continued*

Summary	Indicators	Verification	Assumptions and Risks
1.5 Arrange learning activities; find resources for cover/fees; locate courses			1.5 Appropriate and affordable education and training available, matching learning needs, learning style, time
1.6 Practise and apply new skills			1.6 Have gained sufficient skills from courses attended and other learning to be good enough to practise
1.7 Monitor that learning has taken place/been applied			1.7 Know how and have skills to assess own role in delivery and quality of care and services Risk might be:
1.8 Get course curriculum and talk to someone who has been to proposed training course			1.8 Selected course is inappropriate for you
1.9 Discuss your PDP with peer to look at gaps you have not recognised			
2.1 Be familiar with clinical governance plan and NHS priorities			2.1 Understand components of clinical governance
2.2 Link own work to clinical governance plan			2.2 Own work is congruent with clinical governance plan and can link in
2.3 Make changes to systems and procedures from PDP and clinical governance plan			2.3 Sufficient resources available to enable changes to be made in response to PDP and clinical governance
2.4 Be familiar with requirements for appraisal paperwork and portfolio			2.4 Stay up to date with any revisions to requirements
2.5 Keep records of practice/team's performance			2.5 Make time and capacity for record-keeping; able to distinguish individual's from team's performance
2.6 Compile appraisal portfolio and regularly update it			2.6 Can make time to keep portfolio updated; others supply essential information about your practice or performance

continued overleaf

Table 15.5: *continued*

Summary	Indicators	Verification	Assumptions and Risks
2.7 Submit appraisal portfolio and paperwork to appraiser			2.7 Know who appraiser is in good time; agreed format of appraisal paperwork Risk might be:
2.8 Convene a meeting of managers and practitioners where priorities for clinical governance are thrashed out and consensus reached **2.9 Discuss your evolving PDP with colleagues and staff to determine and agree the implications for their workload and roles**			2.8 PCO/hospital management have different priorities to you and other practitioners for clinical governance plan
3.1 Arrange time/ location for appraisal with appraiser			3.1 Can book mutually agreed time and site for appraisal; other diary commitments do not mean postponements
3.2 Arrange cover for appraisal			3.2 Able to cancel booked surgery or outpatient clinic or find locum cover
3.3 Ensure no interruptions while appraisal takes place			3.3 Appraiser and appraisee both able to arrange for emergencies to be covered by others; able to find quiet room for appraisal
3.4 Prepare well for appraisal – reflect on gaps and plans			3.4 PCO and hospital trust supply information about own practice and performance in good time; have opportunity to reflect on own performance; able to recognise gaps Risks might be:
3.5 Arrange alternative cross-cover from colleague to cover emergency if let down by current arrangements			3.5 Locum who arranged to cover your work is ill and cannot work

continued opposite

Table 15.5: *continued*

	Summary	Indicators	Verification	Assumptions and Risks
	3.6 Become familiar with the appeals process if you/appraiser disagree about the expectations or outcome of your PDP or the appraisal itself			
	4.1 Evolve a culture of mutual support between colleagues to gain cross-cover or another locum			

Now it is time to map out the assumptions and risks associated with your purpose and overall goal. We have started this process with the additions in **bold** in Table 15.6, but in reality you would have far more to add in these sections. You need to think of any external factors that are needed or that might prevent the long-term sustainability of your goal or purpose for the project to be successful. Doctors and others have difficulty differentiating appraisal, which is educational and developmental, from revalidation, which is about assessing that a doctor meets minimum standards of practice, and at the same time accepting that five appraisals can be central to a revalidation portfolio. Thus, although we may assume that the relationship between appraisal and revalidation remains as described, there is a risk that appraisal becomes more of an assessment process over time.

You will need to think about the 'potential risks' that are likely to arise too. The assumptions that you are making and the risks you anticipate should trigger you to add extra activities and outputs to your right-hand column in real life. We have *not* added any extra activities or outputs here in our example log frame in Table 15.6 for the sake of simplicity, but you will certainly have to do so to take adequate measures to ensure your smooth progress with your plan.

Your final step will be to describe the indicators for all your activities, outputs, purpose and goal – and the means by which you can verify that you have achieved them. You should add a timescale too for each indicator.

The indicators should be achievable and worthwhile.

Table 15.6: Step 6 of building up the log frame to achieve successful appraisals and ultimately revalidation – adding various assumptions that you are making about your purpose and goal

	Summary	*Indicators*	*Verification*	*Assumptions and Risks*
Goal	1 To achieve successful revalidation			**Assumes that:** **1.1 The General Medical Council/UK government continue to require revalidation in similar format** **1.2 You remain working in the health service and do not have significant breaks of service** **Risk may be that:** **1.3 Other significant life events occur e.g. you become physically disabled and unable to use your skills**
Purpose	1 Successful appraisal each year			**Assumes that:** **1.1 Five-yearly appraisals continue to be central to revalidation portfolio** **1.2 You have the resources to implement the programme and systems agreed at subsequent appraisals** **Risk may be that:** **1.3 Your PCO/hospital trust change their requirements for appraisal e.g. extent of information reported to management which creates a secretive and defensive culture among participating doctors**
Outputs (intermediate achievements)	1 Action from previous PDP successfully concluded			Assumes that: 1.1 You identified key areas about which you needed to learn more 1.2 You have applied your new knowledge and skills consistently

continued opposite

Table 15.6: *continued*

	Summary	Indicators	Verification	Assumptions and Risks
				1.3 You recognise how your applying learning and changing the way you practise impinges on other team members
				Risk might be that:
				1.4 You have blind spots about the contents of your PDP or the way you have applied your learning
	2 Appraisal portfolio approved by appraiser and PCO or hospital management			2.1 Your appraiser is competent to recognise good practice within appraisal portfolio and PDP
				2.2 Decision by which appraiser rates your appraisal portfolio is fair and transparent
				Risk might be that:
				2.3 Colleagues and/or staff are not agreeable to change their responsibilities or for their job descriptions to be revised
	3 Successful appraisal interview			3.1 Your appraiser is competent to run the appraisal in a constructive way
				Risk might be that:
				3.2 The appraisee and appraiser disagree about the way that plans agreed at previous appraisal have been carried out, or about extent to which limited resources have impeded progress or future priorities
Activities				Assumes that:
	1.1 Identify learning needs			1.1 Know how and have skills to undertake learning needs assessment
	1.2 Seek patient feedback about own work			1.2 Know how and have skills to seek patient feedback

continued overleaf

Table 15.6: *continued*

Summary	Indicators	Verification	Assumptions and Risks
1.3 Understand meaning of seven headings in *GMP*			1.3 Headings in *GMP* are unambiguous and interpreted in same way by all
1.4 Prioritise learning needs and compose PDP			1.4 Know how to prioritise needs and draw up PDP
1.5 Arrange learning activities; find resources for cover/fees; locate courses			1.5 Appropriate and affordable education and training available, matching learning needs, learning style, time
1.6 Practise and apply new skills			1.6 Have gained sufficient skills from courses attended and other learning to be good enough to practise
1.7 Monitor that learning has taken place/been applied			1.7 Know how and have skills to assess own role in delivery and quality of care and services Risk might be:
1.8 Get course curriculum and talk to someone who has been to proposed training course			1.8 Selected course is inappropriate for you
1.9 Discuss your PDP with peer to look at gaps you have not recognised			
2.1 Be familiar with clinical governance plan and NHS priorities			2.1 Understand components of clinical governance
2.2 Link own work to clinical governance plan			2.2 Own work is congruent with clinical governance plan and can link in
2.3 Make changes to systems and procedures from PDP and clinical governance plan			2.3 Sufficient resources available to enable changes to be made in response to PDP and clinical governance
2.4 Be familiar with requirements for appraisal paperwork and portfolio			2.4 Stay up to date with any revisions to requirements

continued opposite

Table 15.6: *continued*

Summary	Indicators	Verification	Assumptions and Risks
2.5 Keep records of practice/team's performance			2.5 Make time and capacity for record-keeping; able to distinguish individual's from team's performance
2.6 Compile appraisal portfolio and regularly update it			2.6 Can make time to keep portfolio updated; others supply essential information about your practice or performance
2.7 Submit appraisal portfolio and paperwork to appraiser			2.7 Know who appraiser is in good time; agreed format of appraisal paperwork Risk might be:
2.8 Convene a meeting of managers and practitioners where priorities for clinical governance are thrashed out and consensus reached			2.8 PCO/hospital management have different priorities to you and other practitioners for clinical governance plan
2.9 Discuss your evolving PDP with colleagues and staff to determine and agree the implications for their workload and roles			
3.1 Arrange time/ location for appraisal with appraiser			3.1 Can book mutually agreed time and site for appraisal; other diary commitments do not mean postponements
3.2 Arrange cover for appraisal			3.2 Able to cancel booked surgery or outpatient clinic or find locum cover
3.3 Ensure no interruptions while appraisal takes place			3.3 Appraiser and appraisee both able to arrange for emergencies to be covered by others; able to find quiet room for appraisal

continued overleaf

Table 15.6: *continued*

	Summary	*Indicators*	*Verification*	*Assumptions and Risks*
	3.4 Prepare well for appraisal – reflect on gaps and plans			3.4 PCO and hospital trust supply information about own practice and performance in good time; have opportunity to reflect on own performance; able to recognise gaps
				Risks might be:
	3.5 Arrange alternative cross-cover from colleague to cover emergency if let down by current arrangements			3.5 Locum who arranged to cover your work is ill and cannot work
	3.6 Become familiar with the appeals process if you/appraiser disagree about the expectations or outcome of your PDP or the appraisal itself			
	4.1 Evolve a culture of mutual support between colleagues to gain cross-cover or another locum			
	You will add other activities and outputs to address the assumptions and risks you have just included in the purpose and goal sections			

Table 15.7: Step 7 of building up the log frame to achieve successful appraisals and ultimately revalidation – adding indicators and the means of verification of progress for your planned activities, outputs, purpose and goal

	Summary	*Indicators (examples)*	*Verification (examples)*	*Assumptions and Risks*
Goal	1 To achieve successful revalidation	**Revalidation portfolio including reports from five annual appraisals is submitted on time, five-yearly**	**Revalidation group agree portfolio is of the required standard every five years**	**As for Table 15.6**
Purpose	1 Successful appraisal each year	**1.1 Appraiser approves standards of appraisal portfolio and satisfactory discussion, annually** **1.2 PCO/ hospital accept appraiser's report of satisfactory appraisal, annually**	**1.1 Written report by appraiser(s) confirms appraisee has reached a satisfactory standard, annually** **1.2 PCO/ hospital management issue written confirmation of appraiser's verdict, annually**	**As for Table 15.6**
Outputs (intermediate achievements)	1 Action from previous PDP successfully concluded	**1.1 Record of learning in revised PDP for current year shows progression from previous action plan**	**1.1 Appraiser's report accepts that completion of previous year's PDP has been satisfactory**	**As for Table 15.6**
	2 Appraisal portfolio approved by appraiser and PCO or hospital management	**2.1 Appraiser approves standards of appraisal portfolio**	**2.1 Written report by appraiser(s) confirms appraisal portfolio is of a satisfactory standard**	

continued overleaf

Table 15.7: *continued*

Summary	Indicators (examples)	Verification (examples)	Assumptions and Risks
	2.2 PCO/ hospital accept appraiser's report of satisfactory appraisal	**2.2 PCO/ hospital management issue written confirmation of appraiser's verdict**	**As for Table 15.6**
3 Successful appraisal interview	**3.1 Constructive discussion**	**3.1 Appraisee values the appraisal interview in subsequent evaluation**	
	3.2 Consensus reached about action plan for coming year by appraiser/ appraisee	**3.2 Appraiser and appraisee both sign the report of the outcomes of the appraisal before it is sent to PCO/hospital management**	
Activities	1.1 Identify learning needs	**1.1 Learning needs exercises carried out by x months**	**1.1 At least two types of exercises undertaken giving objective data about performance**	**As for Table 15.6**
	1.2 Seek patient feedback about own work	**1.2 Patients' views sought by x months and responded to by y months**	**1.2 Validated method of obtaining patients' views used. Subsequent review demonstrates response made to patients' views**	

continued opposite

Table 15.7: *continued*

Summary	Indicators (examples)	Verification (examples)	Assumptions and Risks
1.3 Understand meaning of seven headings in *GMP*	**1.3 Appraisal portfolio arranged under section headings of *GMP* by end of year**	**1.3 Appraiser's report confirms that appraisee has demonstrated that s/he is above minimum standards in these seven areas**	
1.4 Prioritise learning needs and compose PDP	**1.4 PDP drawn up, based upon priority needs by x months**	**1.4 Appraiser's written report confirms that current PDP framework is satisfactory**	
1.5 Arrange learning activities; find resources for cover/fees; locate courses	**1.5 Undertaken planned activities by x months**	**1.5 Appraiser's written report confirms that previous PDP has been undertaken satisfactorily**	
1.6 Practise and apply new skills	**1.6 Quality indicators relating to new skills are met by x months**	**1.6 Audit of quality indicators confirms new skills are safely integrated into everyday practice**	
1.7 Monitor that learning has taken place/been applied	**1.7 Audit learning in topic and that it has been applied in practice by x months**	**1.7 Audit of practice confirms that learning has led to appropriate changes being made**	
1.8 Get course curriculum and talk to someone who has been to proposed training course	**1.8 Discuss course curriculum with previous participant**	**1.8 Copy of course curriculum/ discussion takes place**	

continued overleaf

Table 15.7: *continued*

Summary	Indicators (examples)	Verification (examples)	Assumptions and Risks
1.9 Discuss your PDP with peer to look at gaps you have not recognised	**1.9 Discussion of PDP with peer**	**1.9 Previously unrecognised weaknesses of PDP identified by discussion with peer**	
2.1 Be familiar with clinical governance plan and NHS priorities	**2.1 Know how NHS priorities affect clinical governance plan**	**2.1 Include clinical governance plan/list of relevant NHS priorities in appraisal documentation**	
2.2 Link own work to clinical governance plan	**2.2 Overlap priorities in own PDP and work plan with clinical governance plan**	**2.2 Identify links of own work with NHS priorities and clinical governance plan in appraisal portfolio**	
2.3 Make changes to systems and procedures at work	**2.3 Make changes to systems and procedures from PDP and clinical governance plan by x months**	**2.3 Changes made are demonstrably important for patient care**	
2.4 Be familiar with requirements for appraisal paperwork and portfolio	**2.4 Can explain contents of appraisal paperwork and portfolio to another person**	**2.4 Example of explanation of appraisal paperwork/ portfolio to other person e.g. colleague, junior staff**	
2.5 Records practice/team's performance	**2.5 Keep record of how team perform at least at acceptable standard**	**2.5 Keep record of how team perform at least at acceptable standard in key topic areas**	

continued opposite

Table 15.7: *continued*

Summary	Indicators (examples)	Verification (examples)	Assumptions and Risks
2.6 Compile appraisal portfolio and regularly update it	**2.6 Appraisal portfolio updated at least quarterly**	**2.6 Appraisal portfolio approved by appraiser at annual appraisal or interim review**	
2.7 Submit appraisal portfolio and paperwork to appraiser	**2.7 Appraisal paperwork/ portfolio submitted at least three weeks before appraisal**	**2.7 Appraiser received appraisal portfolio and completed paperwork**	
2.8 Convene a meeting of managers and practitioners where priorities for clinical governance are thrashed out and consensus reached	**2.8 Meeting held and consensus reached by x months**	**2.8 Team meeting attended by key managers and practitioners; all agree outcome**	
2.9 Discuss your evolving PDP with colleagues and staff to determine and agree the implications for their workload and roles	**2.9 Your PDP is discussed with others in team**	**2.9 Your PDP fits within the overall workforce development plan for your practice, directorate or trust**	
3.1 Arrange time/ location for appraisal with appraiser	**3.1 Appraisal meeting arranged at mutually convenient time/ site**	**3.1 Appraisal meeting booked in appraiser's and appraisee's diaries**	
3.2 Arrange cover for appraisal	**3.2 Cover arranged in good time**	**3.2 Your colleagues/ manager know details of your cover arrangements**	

continued overleaf

Table 15.7: *continued*

	Summary	Indicators (examples)	Verification (examples)	Assumptions and Risks
	3.3 Ensure no interruptions while appraisal takes place	**3.3 Place notice outside appraisal interview room and stop incoming phone calls**	**3.3 No interruptions occur while appraisal underway**	
	3.4 Prepare well for appraisal – reflect on gaps and plans	**3.4 Appraisal portfolio submitted in good time; spend appropriate time reflecting on forthcoming appraisal**	**3.4 There are no surprises at appraisal interview that you could have predicted if you had prepared more effectively**	
	3.5 Arrange alternative cross-cover from colleague to cover emergency if let down by current arrangements	**3.5 Make alternative cross-cover arrangements for time of appraisal**	**3.5 Your colleagues/ manager know details of your alternative cover arrangements**	
	3.6 Become familiar with the appeals process if you/appraiser disagree about the expectations or outcome of your PDP or the appraisal itself	**3.6 Know details of appeals process**	**3.6 Give colleagues details of the appeals process**	
	4.1 Evolve a culture of mutual support between colleagues to gain cross-cover or another locum	**4.1 Establish opportunities to share problems and offer support**	**4.1 Colleague(s) volunteer to provide cross-cover during your appraisal or at other time**	

Concluding your logical plan

Now that you have finished mapping out your log frame, you should refine it and maybe discuss it with someone else to see if it is realistic or if there is something else that you have not thought of.

Decide how often you are going to review it. A six-monthly review, say, should enable you to keep a track of your progress with your project. The extent to which you meet the indicators should give you a good idea about how you are getting on. You may then realise, too, that there are additional assumptions and risks that you have not previously thought of or addressed.

References

1   Coleman G (1987) Logical framework approach to the monitoring and evaluation of agricultural and rural development projects. *Project Appraisal.* **2(4)**: 251–9.

2   Centre for Rural Development and Training (2000) *A Guide for Developing a Logical Framework.* University of Wolverhampton, Wolverhampton.

3   Spender A and Chambers R (2002) *Logical Framework for the Teenwise Project.* Staffordshire University, Stoke-on-Trent.

APPENDIX 1

Sources of information and help

Websites

- **American Board of Internal Medicine** www.abim.org
- **American College of Physicians and American Society of Internal Medicine** www.acponline.org/public/bedside/?idx
- **British Association of Medical Managers** www.bamm.co.uk
- **British Medical Association (BMA)** www.bma.org.uk/ap.nsf/Content/_Home_Public
- **Department of Health (DoH)** www.doh.gov.uk/gpappraisal/
- **Edgecumbe Consulting Group Ltd** www.edgecumbe.com
- **EQUIP (Educational organisation for North Essex)** www.equip.ac.uk/cgi/equip/title.php3
- **General Medical Council (GMC)** www.revalidationuk.info/
- **National Association of Non-Principals (NANP)** www.nanp.org.uk
- **National Electronic Library of Medicine** www.nelh.nhs.uk
- **NHS appraisal** www.doh.gov.uk/gpappraisal
- **NHS appraisals toolkit (Sowerby Centre for Health Informatics at Newcastle [SCHIN])** www.appraisals.nhs.uk
- **Royal College of General Practitioners (RCGP)** www.rcgp.org.uk/
- **School of Health and Related Research (ScHARR)** www.shef.ac.uk/~scharr
- **TRIP database** www.tripdatabase.com

Further reading

- British Association of Medical Managers (1999) *Appraisal in Action.* British Association of Medical Managers, Stockport.

- Chambers R (ed.) (2002) *A Guide to Accredited Professional Development: modules file.* Royal College of General Practitioners, London.

- Chambers R (ed.) (2002) *A Guide to Accredited Professional Development: pathway to revalidation.* Royal College of General Practitioners, London.

- Chambers R and Wall D (2000) *Teaching Made Easy; a manual for health professionals.* Radcliffe Medical Press, Oxford.

- Edis M (1995) *Performance Management and Appraisal in the Health Services.* Kogan Page, London.

- Gatrell J and White T (2001) *Medical Appraisal, Selection and Revalidation – a professional's guide to good practice.* Royal Society of Medicine, London.

- Haman H, Irvine S and Jelley D (2001) *The Peer Appraisal Handbook for General Practitioners.* Radcliffe Medical Press, Oxford.

- Martin D, Harrison P, Joesbury H *et al.* (2001) *Appraisal for GPs.* School of Health and Related Research, University of Sheffield. Available from Department of Health at www.doh.gov.uk/pricare/gpappraisal.htm.

- Meagher T, Smith R, Bradley R *et al.* (2002) Consultant assessment and appraisal: an outline in practice. *Clin Radiol.* **57 (1)**: 37–40.

- Peyton JWR (2000) *Appraisal and Assessment in Medical Practice.* Manticore Europe Ltd, Rickmansworth.

- Robinson P and Simpson L (2003) *e-Appraisal, a Guide for Primary Care.* Radcliffe Medical Press, Oxford.

- Wilkins S and Matheson K (2001) *Appraisal for Medical Consultants – a handbook of best practice.* Earlybrave Publications Ltd, United Kingdom.

The Accredited Professional Development (APD) programme for GPs

The programme has been developed by the Royal College of General Practitioners (RCGP) in partnership with the Medical Defence Union (MDU). APD is for all GPs in the UK – GP principals or non-principals, members and non-members of the RCGP. APD covers almost all the requirements for annual appraisal and revalidation.

The APD programme is run over a five-year cycle. Module 1 is a continuous module that GPs undertake all the time. The other five modules are rotated over the five-year programme of APD. These encompass: Communication, Medical Record-keeping, Access and Teamworking, Prescribing and Referrals, Complaints and Removals.

Just as for a personal development plan (PDP), GPs assess their personal and professional learning needs, develop and implement a learning plan, and evaluate and reflect on the outcomes. However, with APD they plan this learning cycle around the criteria that describe an 'excellent GP' taken from *Good Medical Practice for General Practitioners*, the document written by the RCGP and the General Practitioners Committee (GPC) that translates the General Medical Council's *Good Medical Practice* into a general practice context. They also involve the rest of their team whenever appropriate.

Options are the APD materials for self-directed use by the GP; or register for an accredited programme facilitated by experienced doctors.

For queries about APD programmes or materials, email: apd@rcgp.org.uk.

To purchase APD materials contact Radcliffe Medical Press. Tel: 01235 528820. Email: education@radcliffemed.com.

APPENDIX 2

Examples of appraisal paperwork

Example 1: Appraisal paperwork for general practitioners working in the NHS in England (forms in brief)

You can download a full set of paperwork from www.doh.gov.uk/gpappraisal.
   There are five forms. The first three are completed by the appraisee before the appraisal discussion:

- Form 1 – basic details.
- Form 2 – current medical activities.
- Form 3 – material for appraisal.

The appraiser will bring two further forms to the appraisal meeting.

- Form 4 – summary of the appraisal (completed during and immediately after the appraisal discussion).
- Form 5 – confidential record of the appraisal discussion.

Form 1: basic details

- Name.
- Registered address and telephone number.
- Main practice address and telephone number.
- Qualifications in UK or elsewhere, with dates.
- GMC registration type currently held, registration number and date of first full registration.
- Date of last revalidation.
- Date of certification as a GP: Joint Committee on Postgraduate Training for General Practice (JCPTGP) certificate or date of starting practice if before 1981.

- Date of appointment to current post if different.
- Main current post in general practice, e.g. General Medical Services (GMS) principal or Personal Medical Services (PMS) doctor with a patient list.
- Other current posts and appointments with (1) starting dates, (2) average time spent on them, (3) whether public sector, such as working for the Benefits Agency, or private sector such as working in a nursing home.
- Previous posts in NHS and elsewhere, in last five years, with dates.
- Other relevant personal details and brief information you wish to record that helps to describe you, e.g. membership of professional groups or societies.

Form 2: current medical activities

This form requires a brief and factual description of the work you do in the practice and in other posts, including:

- a summary of the activities you undertake in your practice during normal working hours, e.g. minor surgery, child health services
- emergency, on-call and out-of-hours work
- brief details of other clinical work, e.g. as clinical assistant, hospital practitioner etc.
- any other NHS or non-NHS work that you undertake as a GP, e.g. teaching, management, research, being an examiner, forensic work
- work for regional, national or international organisations
- other professional activities.

Form 3: material for appraisal

The third form is the one that will require most of your preparation time. You can collect much of this information as you work through Chapters 6 to 15 in the second part of this book – so don't despair.

This form is organised around the core headings used by the General Medical Council in *Good Medical Practice*, and the Royal College of General Practitioners/General Practitioners Committee in *Good Medical Practice for General Practitioners*.[1,2] These same headings will be used to summarise your appraisal discussion.

The nine areas covered in Form 3 tie in with the requirements for revalidation.

1   Good clinical care (*see* Chapter 6).
2   Maintaining good medical practice (*see* Chapter 7).
3   Relationships with patients (*see* Chapter 8).

4　Working with colleagues (*see* Chapter 9).
5　Teaching and training (*see* Chapter 10).
6　Probity (*see* Chapter 11).
7　Management activity (*see* Chapter 12).
8　Research (*see* Chapter 13).
9　Health (*see* Chapter 14).

You will be filling in information within these nine areas about:

- what you do now
- how you have improved since your last appraisal
- what you think, or have established, that you need to do to improve – this will include your continuing development needs
- what stops you doing as well as you would like to do
- how you see your job and career developing over the next few years
- any health-related issues that may put patients at risk
- overview of development, development needs, constraints during the year.

Then sign the completed form as an accurate report, along with the appraiser.

Form 4: summary of the appraisal and personal development plan

Your appraisal folder should include a summary of your last appraisal and what you have since achieved in your last personal development plan (that is, last year's Form 4 if you have had a previous appraisal).

Form 4 starts with a summary of the appraisal discussion in the following areas.

- Good clinical care.
- Maintaining good medical practice.
- Relationships with patients.
- Working with colleagues.
- Teaching and training.
- Probity.
- Management activity.
- Research.
- Health.
- Any other points.

You then proceed to your personal development plan (PDP). You may well have your own style of PDP. Make sure that it contains the same sections as are within the official version in the appraisal paperwork so that they overlap and you do not have to rewrite your PDP for your appraisal. If you are unsure how to identify any part of your PDP cycle, you can find useful information about each of these stages in other books.[3,4] The column headings in this plan are as follows.

- What development needs do I have?
- How will I address them?
- Date by which I plan to achieve the development goal.
- Outcome.
- Completed.

This form is again signed by both appraiser and appraisee.

Form 5: detailed confidential account of appraisal interview

This form provides an optional framework for keeping a fuller account of the appraisal discussion. It has similar section headings to those of Forms 3 and 4. It is confidential in that it is not intended to be sent to the clinical governance lead and chief executive of the primary care trust as the other Forms 1 to 4 are.

This form is again signed by both appraiser and appraisee.

Example 2: Appraisal paperwork for consultants working in the NHS in England (forms in brief)

You can download a full set of paperwork from www.revalidationuk.info/.

There are six forms. The appraisee should complete the first three forms prior to the appraisal meeting.

- Form 1 – background details.
- Form 2 – current medical activities.
- Form 3 – material for appraisal.

The three further forms completed at the appraisal discussion or immediately afterwards are as follows.

- Form 4 – summary of appraisal discussion (completed by appraiser and agreed by the appraisee) + personal development plan.
- Form 5 – personal and organisational effectiveness.
- Form 6 – confidential record of appraisal interview.

Form 1: background details

- Name.
- Registered address (and contact address if different).
- Main employer.
- Other employers/places of work.
- Date of primary medical or dental qualification (in the UK or elsewhere).
- GMC registration (type of registration currently held, registration number and date of first full registration).
- Starting date of first appointment as a substantive consultant in the NHS, including honorary appointment.
- Date of appointment to post currently held, if different.
- Title of post currently held.
- Date and country of grant of any specialist registration/qualification outside the UK and specialty in which you were registered.
- Any other specialties or sub-specialties in which you are registered.
- Has your registration been called into question since your last appraisal? (If this is the first appraisal, is your registration currently in question?)
- Date of last revalidation (if applicable).
- All the posts in which you have been employed (including honorary and part-time posts) in the NHS and elsewhere in the past five years.
- Other relevant personal details.

Form 2: current medical activities

This form provides an opportunity to describe your post(s) in the NHS, in other public sector bodies, or in the private sector, including titles and grades of any posts currently held, or held in the past year. You should detail:

- factors which you believe affect the provision of good healthcare, including your views (supported by information and evidence) on the resources available
- action taken by you to address any obstacles to the provision of good healthcare.

You should keep a copy of your job plan in this section of your folder.

Form 3: record of reference documentation supporting the appraisal and report on development action in the past year

The aim of Form 3 is to provide any background evidence and information that will help to inform your appraisal discussions in the terms set out in the GMC's *Good Medical Practice*. You should also set out your personal development activity for the past year.

You should do this for all fields of practice within which you work for the NHS and outside the NHS.

Record of reference documentation: good medical practice

1 GOOD MEDICAL CARE

Examples of documentation which may be appropriate:

- current job plan/work programme
- indicative information regarding annual caseload/workload
- up-to-date audit data
- record of how results of audit have resulted in changes to practice (if applicable) and other routine indicators of the standards of your care which you yourself use.

2 MAINTAINING GOOD MEDICAL PRACTICE

The purpose of this section is to record continuing professional development (CPD)/continuing medical education (CME) activities undertaken since the last appraisal. Any difficulties in attending should be recorded, with reasons. Examples of documentation should be included and a list of all CPD courses attended, and points awarded for each attendance.

3 WORKING RELATIONSHIPS WITH COLLEAGUES

Examples of documentation which may be appropriate:

- a description of the setting within which you work and the team structure within which you practise
- any other documentary evidence that may be available (such as records of any formal peer reviews or discussions).

4 RELATIONS WITH PATIENTS

Examples of documentation which may be appropriate:

- any examples of good practice or concern in your relationships with patients
- a description of your approach to handling informed consent.

This might include validated patients' surveys, your assessment of any changes in your practice as a result of any investigated complaint, compliments from patients, peer reviews/surveys.

5 TEACHING AND TRAINING

Any difficulties in arranging cover for your clinical work while undertaking teaching and training (including educational activities for the NHS generally) should be recorded.

Examples of documentation which may be appropriate:

- a summary of formal teaching/lecturing activities, supervision/mentoring duties, any recorded feedback from those taught.

6 PROBITY AND 7 HEALTH

These sections give you the opportunity to record any concerns raised or problems encountered during the year on either of these issues and include any records.

8 MANAGEMENT ACTIVITY

Examples of documentation which may be appropriate:

- information about your formal management commitments, records of any noteworthy achievements and any recorded feedback if available.

You can add any further information, including any difficulties in arranging cover for your clinical work while undertaking local or national management activity.

9 RESEARCH

Examples of documentation which may be appropriate:

- evidence of formal research commitments
- record of any research ongoing or completed in the previous year
- record of noteworthy achievements
- confirmation that appropriate ethical approval has been secured for all research undertaken.

REPORT ON DEVELOPMENT ACTION IN THE PAST YEAR

You should summarise here the development action agreed at the last appraisal (or at any interim meeting) or include your personal development plan. You should record where it is agreed that goals have been achieved or where further action is required. A development need that has not been met in full will remain a need and will either be reflected in the coming year's plan or have resulted in other action.

This form is signed by both appraiser and appraisee.

Form 4: summary of appraisal discussion with agreed action and personal development plan

The aim of this form is to provide an agreed summary of the appraisal discussion based on the documents listed in Form 3 and a description of the action agreed in the course of the appraisal, including those forming the personal development plan.

Form 4 starts with a summary of the appraisal discussion in the following areas.

- Good medical care.
- Maintaining good medical practice.
- Working relationships with colleagues.
- Relationships with patients.
- Teaching and training.
- Probity.
- Health.
- Any other points.

This form should be completed by the appraiser and agreed by the appraisee. Under each heading the appraiser should explain which of the documents listed in Form 3 informed this part of the discussion, the conclusion reached and say what, if any, action has been agreed.

Personal development plan

The appraiser and appraisee should identify key development objectives for the year ahead, which relate to the appraisee's personal and/or professional development. This will include action identified in the summary above but may also include other development activity. The timescales should be clearly indicated.

The important areas to cover are:

- action to maintain skills and the level of service to patients
- action to develop or acquire new skills
- action to change or improve existing practice.

If you are unsure how to identify any part of your personal development plan cycle, you can find useful information about each of these stages in other books.[3,4] The column headings in this plan are as follows.

- What development needs do I have?
- How will I address them?
- Date by which I plan to achieve the development goal.

- Outcome.
- Completed.

This form is again signed by both appraiser and appraisee.

Form 5: personal and organisational effectiveness

The aim of this form is to describe your effectiveness on a personal level and within the NHS organisation where you work, with a view to informing job plan review. For example:

- the contribution you make to the development of services
- the delivery of service outcomes
- your identification of the resources needed to improve personal effectiveness.

The appraiser should prepare a workload summary with the appraisee.
    Examples of documentation which may be appropriate:

- agreed service-related objectives and work programme (if not included elsewhere)
- relevant comparative performance data
- any advice from the appropriate royal college, faculty or specialty association on workload or productivity
- nationally or locally agreed comparators or performance standards
- any local policies, goals or service standards which influence or affect performance
- a note of any difficulties you may have had in obtaining your entitlements to annual leave etc.
- a note of any changes in the job plan proposed either by the appraisee or the appraiser.

This form is again signed by both appraiser and appraisee.

Form 6: detailed confidential account of appraisal interview

This form is available to provide the opportunity, if required, to record a fuller, more detailed account of the appraisal discussion than is recorded on Form 4. It is not obligatory. Form 6 is confidential and is not intended to form part of the documentation going to the chief executive.
    It is set out under the seven main headings of *Good Medical Practice.*[1]
    This form is again signed by both appraiser and appraisee.

References

1   General Medical Council (2001) *Good Medical Practice.* General Medical Council, London.

2   Royal College of General Practitioners/General Practitioners Committee (2002) *Good Medical Practice for General Practitioners.* Royal College of General Practitioners, London.

3   Wakley G, Chambers R and Field S (2000) *Continuing Professional Development in Primary Care: making it happen.* Radcliffe Medical Press, Oxford.

4   Rughani A (2000) *The GP's Guide to Personal Development Plans.* Radcliffe Medical Press, Oxford.

APPENDIX 3

Template for a detailed personal development plan (PDP)

This is a more detailed template for a PDP than the format given in the standard appraisal paperwork of Appendix 2. Start with one main topic and add others as you justify needing to learn more about them.

What topic have you chosen?

Why is the topic a priority?

(i) A personal and professional priority?

(ii) A practice or workplace priority?

(iii) A district priority?

(iv) A national priority?

Who will be included in your personal plan?
(Anyone other than you? Other doctors, members of your team, patients?)

What baseline information will you collect and how?

How will you identify your learning needs? How will you obtain this and who will do it?
(Self-completion checklists, discussion, appraisal, audit, patient feedback?)

What are the learning needs for your department or practice and how do they match your needs?

Is there any patient or public input to your personal development plan?

continued overleaf

How might you integrate the 14 components of clinical governance into your personal development plan?

Establishing a learning culture:

Managing resources and services:

Establishing a research and development culture:

Reliable and accurate data:

Evidence-based practice and policy:

Confidentiality:

Health gain:

Coherent team:

Audit and evaluation:

Meaningful involvement of patients and the public:

Health promotion:

Risk management:

Accountability and performance:

Core requirements:

Objectives of your personal development plan arising from the preliminary data-gathering exercise:

Action plan
(Include timetabled action and expected outcomes):

How does your personal development plan tie in with your other strategic plans?

continued opposite

What additional resources will you require to execute your plan and from where do you hope to obtain them?
(Will you have to pay any course fees? Will you be able to organise any protected time for learning in working hours?)

How will you evaluate your personal development plan?

How will you know when you have achieved your objectives?
(How will you measure success?)

How will you disseminate the learning from your plan to the rest of your team and patients? How will you sustain your new-found knowledge or skills?

How will you handle new learning requirements as they crop up?

Record of your learning activities
Write in the topic, date, time spent and type of learning

	Activity 1	Activity 2	Activity 3	Activity 4
In-house formal learning				
External courses				
Informal and personal				
Qualifications and/or experience gained				

Index